Women's Health

Guest Editor

ELLEN OLSHANSKY, DNSc, WHNP-BC, FAAN

NURSING CLINICS
OF NORTH AMERICA

www.nursing.theclinics.com

Consulting Editor
SUZANNE S. PREVOST, RN, PhD, COI

September 2009 • Volume 44 • Number 3

SAUNDERS an imprint of ELSEVIER, Inc.

W.B. SAUNDERS COMPANY

A Division of Elsevier Inc.

1600 John F. Kennedy Blvd., Suite 1800 • Philadelphia, PA 19103-2899

http://www.theclinics.com

NURSING CLINICS OF NORTH AMERICA Volume 44, Number 3
September 2009 ISSN 0029-6465, ISBN-13: 978-1-4377-1247-6, ISBN-10: 1-4377-1247-9

Editor: Katie Hartner
Developmental Editor: Donald Mumford

Nursing Clinics of North America (ISSN 0029-6465) is published quarterly by Elsevier Inc., 360 Park Avenue South, New York, NY 10010-1710. Months of issue are March, June, September, and December. Periodicals postage paid at New York, NY and additional mailing offices. Subscription price per year is, $133.00 (US individuals), $273.00 (US institutions), $228.00 (international individuals), $334.00 (international institutions), $184.00 (Canadian individuals), $334.00 (Canadian institutions), $70.00 (US students), and $115.00 (international students). To receive student/resident rate, orders must be accompanied by name of affiliated institution, date of term, and the signature of program/residency coordinator on institution letterhead. Orders will be billed at individual rate until proof of status is received. Foreign air speed delivery is included in all *Clinics* subscription prices. All prices are subject to change without notice. **POSTMASTER:** Send address changes to *Nursing Clinics*, Elsevier Health Sciences Division, Subscription Customer Service, 3251 Riverport Lane, Maryland Heights, MO 63043. **Customer Service: Telephone: 1-800-654-2452** (U.S. and Canada); **1-314-447-8871** (outside U.S. and Canada). **Fax: 1-314-447-8029. E-mail: journalscustomerservice-usa@elsevier.com** (for print support) and **journalsonlinesupport-usa@elsevier.com** (for online support).

Nursing Clinics of North America is covered in *EMBASE/Excerpta Medica, MEDLINE/PubMed (Index Medicus), Social Sciences Citation Index, Current Contents, ASCA, Cumulative Index to Nursing, RNdex Top 100,* and Allied Health Literature and International Nursing Index (INI).

Printed in the United States of America.

Contributors

CONSULTING EDITOR

SUZANNE S. PREVOST, RN, PhD, COI
Associate Dean, Practice and Community Engagement, University of Kentucky, Lexington, Kentucky

GUEST EDITOR

ELLEN OLSHANSKY, DNSc, WHNP-BC, FAAN
Professor and Director, Program in Nursing Science, College of Health Sciences, University of California, Irvine, California

AUTHORS

JUDITH A. BERG, PhD, RN, WHNP-BC, FAAN, FAANP
Associate Professor, University of Arizona College of Nursing, Tucson, Arizona

LORA E. BURKE, PhD, MPH, FAHA, FAAN
Professor of Nursing and Epidemiology, Department of Health and Community Systems, School of Nursing, Graduate School of Public Health, University of Pittsburgh, Pittsburgh, Pennsylvania

HEIDI DONOVAN, PhD, RN
Assistant Professor, Department of Acute and Tertiary Care, University of Pittsburgh School of Nursing, Pittsburgh, Pennsylvania

PHENSIRI DUMRONGPAKAPAKORN, MSN, RN
Doctoral Student, Department of Acute and Tertiary Care, University of Pittsburgh School of Nursing, Pittsburgh, Pennsylvania

ANASTASIA A. FISHER, RN, DNSc
Associate Professor, School of Nursing, San Francisco State University, San Francisco, California

REBEKAH HAMILTON, PhD, RN
Assistant Professor, Department of Women, Children and Family Health Science, College of Nursing, University of Illinois at Chicago, Chicago, Illinois

DIANE C. HATTON, RN, DNSc
Professor, School of Nursing, San Diego State University, San Diego, California

KATHY HOPKINS, MS, RN
Doctoral Student, Department of Acute and Tertiary Care, University of Pittsburgh School of Nursing, Pittsburgh, Pennsylvania

JANE H. KASS-WOLFF, PhD, FNP, WHNP
Assistant Professor, Women, Children, and Family Health, College of Nursing, University of Colorado Denver, Aurora, Colorado

MARY KNUDTSON, DNSc, NP, FAAN
Professor of Clinical Nursing, Program in Nursing Science, Department of Nursing,
University of California Irvine, Irvine, California

AMY J. LEVI, CNM, PhD, FACNM
Clinical Professor, Department of Obstetrics/Gynecology and Reproductive Sciences,
School of Medicine, University of California San Francisco, San Francisco, California

NANCY K. LOWE, CNM, PhD, FACNM, FAAN
Professor and Chair, Women, Children, and Family Health, College of Nursing, University
of Colorado Denver, Aurora, Colorado

ELLEN OLSHANSKY, DNSc, WHNP-BC, FAAN
Professor and Director, Program in Nursing Science, College of Health Sciences,
University of California, Irvine, California

SUSANNE PHILLIPS, MSN, NP
Associate Clinical Professor, Program in Nursing Science, Department of Nursing,
University of California Irvine, Irvine, California

PAULA SHERWOOD, PhD, RN, CNRN
Assistant Professor, Department of Acute and Tertiary Care, University of Pittsburgh
School of Nursing, Pittsburgh, Pennsylvania

KATHERINE E. SIMMONDS, RNC, MSN, MPH
Clinical Instructor, Graduate Program in Nursing, Massachusetts General Hospital
Institute of Health Professions, Charlestown, Massachusetts

DIANA TAYLOR, RN, PhD, FAAN
Professor Emerita, Department of Family Health Care Nursing, School of Nursing,
University of California San Francisco, San Francisco, California

SUSAN TISO, MN, NP
Associate Clinical Professor, Program in Nursing Science, Department of Nursing,
University of California Irvine, Irvine, California

PATRICIA K. TUITE, MSN, RN
Instructor, Department of Acute and Tertiary Care, School of Nursing, University
of Pittsburgh, Pittsburgh, Pennsylvania

MELANIE WARZISKI TURK, PhD, MSN, RN
Assistant Professor, School of Nursing, Duquesne University, Pittsburgh, Pennsylvania

NANCY FUGATE WOODS, PhD, RN, FAAN
Professor of Family and Child Nursing; and Dean Emeritus, University of Washington
School of Nursing, Seattle, Washington

ROBYNN ZENDER, MS
Research Assistant, Program in Nursing Science, College of Health Sciences, University
of California, Irvine, California

KRISTIN ZORN, MD
Assistant Professor, Department of Obstetrics, Gynecology and Reproductive Sciences,
Division of Gynecology, Magee Women's Hospital, University of Pittsburgh Medical
Center, Pittsburgh, Pennsylvania

Contents

There are more than 12,000 women's health nurse practitioners (WHNPs) currently certified by the National Certification Corporation (NCC) and practicing in a wide range of roles. The purpose of this article is to describe the historical development of the WHNP specialty, and to review the evolution of the specialty from an initially very focused practice in the area of family planning into obstetric and gynecologic care to today's more diffuse role inclusive of primary care. Women's health nurse practitioners must broaden their educational background to include the lifespan of women, not just the reproductive years. With the inclusion of chronic disease management of the middle-aged and elderly woman, WHNPs will provide more comprehensive and integrative health care to women in all areas of the United States.

For the purposes of this article, wellness is defined as an individual's subjective experience of overall life satisfaction in relation to physical, mental, emotional, spiritual, social, economic, occupational, and environmental dimensions. Women's wellness focuses on those aspects of well-being that pertain disproportionately, or solely, to women. Wellness includes but is not limited to physical, emotional and social aspects and disruptions that alter a woman's quality of life, such as reproductive and hormonal issues, bone health, gastrointestinal stress, and urinary incontinence. This article discusses women's wellness through the life span, from preconception through death, and considers the implications of these issues for the nursing profession.

Human papillomavirus (HPV) is the most commonly sexually transmitted infection in the United States. This article gives an overview and discussion of HPV virus types and transmission, and the quadrivalent vaccine now available to protect against it. Included are the nursing implications for the HPV vaccine related to education and counseling of parents, patients, and young adult women regarding HPV vaccination, for whom the vaccine is indicated.

has created new opportunities for educating cancer patients and supporting them to better cope with their disease. This article reviews prior studies of computer-based patient education interventions to identify key intervention components and other factors associated with improved patient outcomes. Opportunities for using computer-based technologies to support women with ovarian cancer are discussed and WRITE Symptoms (a Written Representational Intervention To Ease Symptoms), a web-based, symptom management intervention for women with recurrent ovarian cancer, is introduced.

THE CLINICS ARE NOW AVAILABLE ONLINE!
Access your subscription at:
www.theclinics.com

Preface

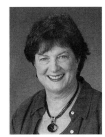

Ellen Olshansky, DNSc, WHNP-BC, FAAN
Guest Editor

As the first decade of the twenty-first century comes to a close, we are faced with many complicated challenges. These are embodied in several critical concerns: the environment, the economy, global relationships, and many others. Health and health care continue to be front and center as major issues of concern. And women's health, in particular, continues to have many unanswered, albeit, important questions. In reality, we can't separate women's health from health in general and we can't separate health from other societal concerns, such as the environment, the economy, and our national and international relationships. All of these aspects comprise the various social determinants of health. We need to understand health within a larger social/economic/cultural context, a context that contains myriad variables that directly affect health. Clearly, women's health overlaps with health in general. Despite this overlap, women's health does contain unique aspects and does deserve special focus. Nurses have carved out an important specialty in women's health. Nurses comprise a significant proportion of health care providers who care for women. In this special issue on women's health, we have strived to present a sample of women's health concerns and to address clinical implications and recommendations based on the current evidence and knowledge available. The intent is to provide the most up-to-date information for nurses who care for women.

The history of nursing and women's health is presented by Kass-Wolff and Lowe. This article includes a historical timeline that emphasizes how the role of the women's health nurse practitioner was developed and continues to develop as an important health care provider for women. This historical perspective lays the foundation for understanding women's health nursing today.

Women suffer from many chronic conditions, such as arthritis, diabetes, cardiovascular disease, and some forms of cancer now considered chronic conditions because of the long-term survival rates for many cancers. This special issue contains information related to promotion of cardiovascular health in an article written by Warzinski,

Nurs Clin N Am 44 (2009) ix–x
doi:10.1016/j.cnur.2009.07.013

Tuite, and Burke. Another article on implications of having a genetic risk for breast cancer is presented by Hamilton. With our increasing scientific knowledge, significant breakthroughs have been achieved in our understanding of genetic predisposition to certain diseases. Such understanding leads to a need to understand the human responses to knowing about one's own genetic risk factors. Ovarian cancer is addressed by Dumrongpakapakorn, Hopkins, Sherwood, Zora, and Donovan, with a focus on the use of computer technology to assist women with ovarian cancer in managing their diagnosis. This article addresses the use of new technology as related to nursing care of women with a complicated life-threatening diagnosis.

A serious health concern falls under the category of sexually transmitted infections. Human papillomavirus is one sexually transmitted infection that has been implicated in cervical cancer. Recently a vaccination to prevent human papillomavirus became available. The evidence to support the efficacy of this vaccine and clinical guidelines for using it are presented by Knudtson, Tiso, and Phillips.

The criminal justice system and its approach to women's health is highlighted in this issue by Fisher and Hatton, who recognize that jails and prisons are the context in which some women live and experience health conditions. Women's health in the criminal justice system poses unique challenges for nursing care. Mental health of women across the lifespan is discussed by Zender and Olshansky, with a particular focus on anxiety and depression.

Reproductive health concerns continue to be a high priority as we address comprehensive women's health and health care. Reproductive health is addressed by Levi, Simmonds, and Taylor, with a focus on the importance of nurses taking an active role in the clinical arena by applying a public health framework.

With our increasingly global context, the health of women must be understood from a global perspective. Berg and Woods address global health of women with a focus on women as caregivers.

With the rising incidence of chronic health conditions in this era of health care reform, it has become ever more important to promote health and prevent those conditions that are preventable. Zender and Olshansky summarize the current state of knowledge related to promoting wellness in women across the lifespan.

Taken together, this compendium of articles is an overview of many, though of course not all, of the contemporary issues related to the health and health care of women, including nurses as key health care providers for women. These articles are intended to capture the current state of the science in these particular areas, to encourage nurses who care for women to continue to seek out ongoing scientific knowledge, to raise questions, and to continually develop effective and high-quality evidence-based practice as they care for women and families.

Ellen Olshansky, DNSc, WHNP-BC, FAAN
Program in Nursing Science
College of Health Sciences
University of California
233 Irvine Hall
Irvine, CA 92697, USA

E-mail address:
e.olshansky@uci.edu (E. Olshansky)

A Historical Perspective of the Women's Health Nurse Practitioner

Jane H. Kass-Wolff, PhD, FNP, WHNP*, Nancy K. Lowe, CNM, PhD, FACNM, FAAN

KEYWORDS

- Women's health • Women's health nurse practitioner
- Training • History • Primary care

Nurse practitioners comprise a significant portion of health care providers in the United States. According to the Health Resources and Services Administration (HRSA),[1] as of 2004 there were an estimated 141,209 nurse practitioners or 8.3% of the registered nurse population, and 77.6% (109,582) are certified as evidenced by successful completion of an examination. This number includes the following specialties: family, adult, pediatric, school health, acute care, and women's health. An estimated 12,000 to 15,000 nurses have completed the educational requirements to become a women's health nurse practitioner (WHNP).[2] Of that number, 12,922 have been certified by the National Certification Corporation as WHNPs and are recognized by state boards of nursing and practice in all 50 states.[3] The purpose of this article is to describe the historical development of the WHNP specialty, and to review the evolution of the specialty from an initially very focused practice in the area of family planning into obstetric and gynecologic care to today's more diffuse role inclusive of primary care. This article includes a brief overview of nursing's involvement in women's health, the women's movement and impetus for family planning services, creation of the role of the WHNP, and the evolution of that role up to the present.

HISTORICAL BACKGROUND

Nursing has been engaged in women's health care since the time of Florence Nightingale whose *Notes on Nursing* detailed the health of women and directed women in caring for loved ones, the injured, or wounded.[4] In the United States women such as Lillian Wald, Margaret Sanger, and Mary Breckinridge identified issues specific to women's health, such as lack of access to care of poor women, lack of control over fertility, and the need for maternity care for women, and developed services directed at women's health issues.[4] The first federal government program for the health care of

---

Women, Children, and Family Health, College of Nursing, University of Colorado Denver, 13120 E, 19th Avenue, Aurora, CO 80045, USA
* Corresponding author.
E-mail address: jane.kass-wolff@ucdenver.edu (J.H. Kass-Wolff).

Nurs Clin N Am 44 (2009) 271–280
doi:10.1016/j.cnur.2009.06.006
0029-6465/09/$ – see front matter © 2009 Elsevier Inc. All rights reserved.
nursing.theclinics.com

women and children was the Sheppard-Towner Maternity and Infancy Act of 1921[5] that provided well child care and maternity services by public health nurses to low-income families. The feminist movement in the 1960s had a profound effect on the advancement of women's health from both a political and health care perspective. Feminists' commitment to equality and nondiscrimination began by placing female sexuality and self-determination at the center of women's health concerns with the publication of *Our Bodies, Ourselves* from the Boston Women's Health Book Collective.[6] Women-specific alternatives including abortion clinics, women-controlled health centers, self-care information and publications, and freestanding birth centers began to flourish in the 1960s and 1970s.[5] During this same time other forces were converging that would open up new advanced practice opportunities for nurses (**Fig. 1**).

Development and approval of the first oral contraceptive, Enovid, in 1960, the intra-uterine device (Lippes Loop) in 1962, and the Dalkon Shield in 1971 allowed women to

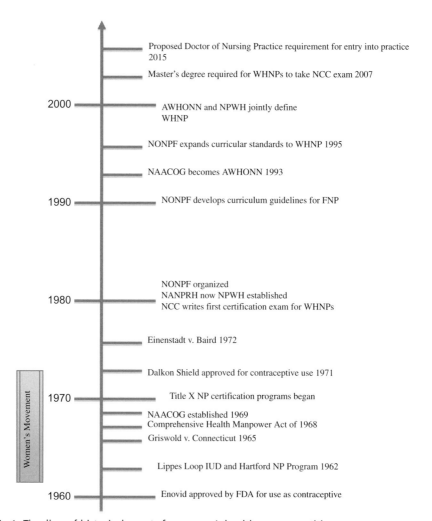

Fig. 1. Timeline of historical events for women's health nurse practitioners.

better control their fertility.[7] Until then most contraceptive methods other than diaphragms were controlled by the woman herself (ie, spermacides, condoms) and did not require the intervention of the physician. This situation changed with the introduction of the birth control pill. Nationwide many states banned the prescription of contraception until the US Supreme Court overturned a lower court decision in *Griswold v. Connecticut* in 1965, allowing married women access to birth control pills.[8] It was not until 1972 that birth control pills were available to unmarried women with the *Eisenstadt v. Baird* decision by the US Supreme Court.[9] This new technology of fertility control required medical supervision; however, the supply and distribution of physicians remained unequal in terms of availability of physicians and access to family planning for women.[7]

During the women's health movement in the 1960s through the 1970s, activists were pivotal in creating awareness of inequities in women's rights, pushing for a comprehensive approach to women's health care and alleviating sexism within the health care system.[10] Nationwide research at this time coincidentally demonstrated disparate access to contraceptives between lower- and higher-income women. Additional research evidence demonstrated that closely spaced pregnancies, either very early or very late in a woman's reproductive years, could have adverse consequences for both mother and child.[11] Unintended pregnancies, particularly in adolescents, limited young women's ability to complete their education, increased their poverty and reliance on public assistance, and limited their participation in the workforce. These findings led to the beginning of a national and governmental movement to improve access to contraception aimed at alleviating poverty and improving the health care of women and children.[11]

Another factor that became obvious during the mid 1960s was the shortage of primary care physicians, particularly in rural and nonmetropolitan areas.[12,13] This phenomenon was related to the fact that a large proportion of physicians chose to specialize rather than remain generalists at a time when access to medical care for all Americans had been broadened, and preventive rather than crisis health care was becoming more accepted.[12] The impetus for the development of the nurse practitioner came first in pediatrics in 1965 at the University of Colorado because of the physician shortage and the simultaneous need to increase access to primary health care, boost the provision of preventive health services, and improve continuity of care for children.[14]

Then in 1972 at the Annual Clinical meeting of the American College of Obstetricians and Gynecologists, a group of physicians and nurses from Hartford Hospital, Connecticut reported on a successful nurse practitioner program in obstetrics and gynecology.[13,14] Hartford Hospital staff had identified similar problems in reproductive health care for women previously noted in children's health care. With the increased complexity and subspecialization within obstetrics and gynecology, the provision of preventive services to women seeking both family planning and obstetric services within their clinics became more problematic for physicians.[14] The role of the nurse practitioner in obstetrics and gynecology was seen as an extension of the role of the nurse but also of the physician. As stated by J. Robert Willson in his inaugural address as president of the American College of Obstetricians and Gynecologists (ACOG) in April 1970: "a competent non-physician associate can do many of the things the obstetrician-gynecologist now does himself, or should do and doesn't".[15]

Hartford Hospital began by developing a nurse specialist program in the labor and delivery unit around 1962. A 16-week program was established that included classroom teaching as well as on-the-job training. Nurses were required to stay at the hospital for 1 year following completion of the training. This program worked so well that the hospital decided to prepare nurses as Family Planning Practitioners to expand services as a part of the ACOG Interconceptional Care Program.[14] Didactic presentations on a variety of topics related to contraception were provided to the nurses along with training to perform physical examinations, including the pelvic examination. The focus of the intensive clinical training was primarily on discerning normal from abnormal, rather than on diagnosis.[14]

DEVELOPMENT PRIOR TO TITLE X FEDERAL FUNDING

Other intensive clinical training programs sprouted up across the country. A contributing factor to the increase in these nurse clinician/nurse practitioner programs was the Comprehensive Health Manpower Act of 1968. This legislation was a continuation and modification of the original Health Professions Educational Assistance Act of 1963, but extended federal assistance to nursing, allied health, and public health professions in the form of loans and scholarships.[16] The intent of this legislation was to expand training facilities and to increase significantly the enrollments within schools training health professionals because of the perceived shortage of primary health care providers that was anticipated in the future. The Comprehensive Health Manpower Act of 1968 served to aid many fledgling nurse practitioner programs. Due to the need for expediency, many of the nurse clinician/nurse practitioner programs developed during this time were brief in length, usually 8-week intensive courses, but with a wide range from 12 days to 24 weeks with either on-the-job training or preceptorships of varying lengths following the intensive classroom program.[12] These programs and their graduates were often not recognized and unregulated by state boards of nursing, with little consistency in curriculum or training and no national certification of the graduates.

Prior to Title X funding, the Planned Parenthood (PP) Federation of America created in-house nurse practitioner programs. Nurses in these programs were trained in 8 weeks to become family planning nurse practitioners (FPNP). There was no prenatal content included in the program, as those services were not provided by PP. On completion of the program, PP certified the nurses to practice as FPNPs. Once Title X programs developed, most states refused to recognize these PP-trained nurse practitioners due to the lack of prenatal care training. To be recognized by the state and to write a certification examination, these nurse practitioners were required to complete the Title X program (Sue Moskosky, personal communication, 2008). Medical schools and nursing and medical schools jointly also began to develop nurse clinician programs to expand their family planning services ranging from 6 to 24 weeks in length.[7] Many nurses working in obstetrics and gynecology also received on-the-job training from physicians (apprenticeship model), and called themselves family planning or obstetric-gynecology (ob-gyn or OGNP) nurse practitioners.[13] There continued to be limited standardization or guidelines for the role or its educational preparation.

DEVELOPMENT AFTER TITLE X FEDERAL FUNDING

As part of the War on Poverty in 1965, the Johnson administration and the federal government through the Office of Economic Opportunity funded the first grants to support the provision of family planning services through programs across the country. Services varied widely from one program to another because states controlled what little funding was available with widely different eligibility criteria and benefit levels.[8,11] That situation changed in 1970 with the enactment of Title X of the Public Health Service (PHS) Act during the Nixon administration. Title X was then and remains the only federal program devoted solely to the provision of family planning services nationwide.[17] By 1972 rules and regulations were promulgated by Congressman George H.W. Bush for the Nixon administration, authorizing grants for projects to provide family planning services to persons from low-income families and other persons desiring those services[8,18] (Sue Moskosky, personal communication, 2008). Under section 1001 of the PHS Act grant monies were authorized to create and establish family planning projects providing a wide range of services that included infertility evaluation, only natural family planning methods, and services to adolescents. Section 1003 of the PHS Act made grants available for the training of family planning practitioners. This last section of Title X provided for the creation of certificate programs for the training of FPNPs across the country.[19]

The certificate programs established by Title X did not support academic programs and could not come under schools of nursing or other academic programs offering degrees. All of the Title X nurse practitioner programs were limited in length to expedite the transition of these nurses back to their work site to provide care with supervision for 9 additional months after the formal program. The initial five programs funded were the University of California Los Angeles-Harbor; the American Federation of Planned Parenthood, New York, that eventually moved to Philadelphia; Emory University in Atlanta, Georgia; Milwaukee Planned Parenthood, Milwaukee, Wisconsin; and the Albuquerque, New Mexico Planned Parenthood. Due to financial issues the grant was taken away from Albuquerque PP and the University of Texas Southwestern Medical School was asked to take over the Title X grant in 1979. Each of the Title X certificate programs drew students from select regions based on public health service areas (Sue Moskosky, personal communication, 2008).

Nurses who worked for Title X grantee organizations (ie, Planned Parenthood, family planning clinics) were given priority in all of the Title X certificate programs, regardless of their level of RN education. Most classes were limited to 10 to 15 students. Students lived in the city where the program was located for 16 weeks of intensive classroom and clinical training that was relatively standardized among the five programs. Training evolved from that of only family planning to include prenatal care. Over the nearly 30 years that the Office of Family Planning in the Office of Population Affairs had oversight of family planning services, more than 5000 family planning and women's health nurse practitioners were prepared in the Title X supported nurse practitioner training.[18] By the late 1990s 80% of the clinicians providing services in Title X clinics were certificate prepared women's health care nurse practitioners. But in the mid 1990s the five certificate programs were having difficulty recruiting trainees, and by 2000 all of the certificate programs were closed due to the high cost of training each student and with the master's degree for entry into practice looming on the horizon. At the same time national organizations and movements within nursing had begun to define the educational requirements and expected competencies for all nurse practitioners, including women's health.

ORGANIZATIONS INFLUENCING THE DEVELOPMENT OF THE WOMEN'S HEALTH NURSE PRACTITIONER

In 1969 the Nurses Association of American College of Obstetricians and Gynecologists (NAACOG) was formed within the American College of Obstetricians and Gynecologists. The association focused on providing educational opportunities and enhancing practice standards for nurses specializing in women's health, obstetric, and neonatal care. In 1972, NAACOG issued a statement on the role of the OGNP.[20] The role was defined as "…a professional practitioner who is capable of

1) collecting significant health data, 2) integrating this information into meaningful assessments, and 3) implementing appropriate therapeutic action on the basis of the above judgments."[20] Collaboration between physician and nurse practitioner was encouraged in the development of management plans for patients, but the OGNP was to manage normal patients and specific abnormal states only after a physician treated abnormal findings that the OGNP identified. Ultimately the physician maintained full responsibility for care provided by the OGNP. In addition, NAACOG determined that the OGNP needed specific training for the role whether in a formal setting or through continuing education.[20] This was the first attempt at describing the role and setting standards for the training of the OGNP. NAACOG separated from the ACOG in 1993 and became the Association of Women's Health, Obstetric and Neonatal Nurses (AWHONN). AWHONN has become a leader in championing women's health issues and has worked to expand the role of the OGNP into the more holistic care role of the WHNP.[21]

In 1980 several events occurred that were to further define the role and describe the training requirements for the obstetric and gynecologic nurse practitioner. The first organizational meeting of the National Organization of Nurse Practitioner Faculties (NONPF) met in Albuquerque, New Mexico.[22] Because of the wide proliferation of all types and varieties of nurse practitioner programs, both certificate and master's level, concern had developed about the dissimilarities in the quality and standards of these programs. In the late 1970s, a National Task Force for Family Nurse Practitioner Curriculum and Evaluation developed guidelines that described 7 domains of practice: (1) management of patient health/illness status; (2) nurse practitioner-patient relationship; (3) teaching-coaching function; (4) professional role; (5) managing and negotiating health care delivery systems; (6) monitoring and ensuring the quality of health care practice; and (7) cultural competence.[23,24] Curricular standards were subsequently expanded to include adult, women's health, and pediatric nurse practitioners. NONPF has continued to focus on preparing quality nurse practitioners through clear guidelines for education.[23]

The National Association of Nurse Practitioners in Reproductive Health, now called the National Association of Nurse Practitioners in Women's Health (NPWH), was established in 1980 to support nurse practitioners in providing quality health care to all women across the lifespan including primary care and specialty practices.[25] In 2000 AWHONN and NPWH jointly defined the WHNP role as follows: "The women's health nurse practitioner provides primary health care to women across the lifespan, with an emphasis on reproductive-gynecologic health. The practitioner uses the processes of assessment, diagnosis, management and evaluation to provide care that integrates the psychosocial and physical needs of women".[26] The focus of the role has broadened to include primary care and a more holistic view of women.

Another significant event was the decision to develop a certification examination for the OGNP or WHNP. The purpose of certification examinations originally was to recognize excellence in practice and the process of seeking certification was strictly voluntary on the part of the nurse.[13] The NAACOG Certification Corporation, now the National Certification Corporation, developed examinations in obstetric and neonatal nursing in the 1970s and in 1980 offered the first certification examination for OGNPs. Although some states required certification by a national professional body as one requirement for state authorization to practice as an advanced practice nurse, most did not. In the mid 1990s the National Council of State Boards of Nursing (NCSBN) became aware that there was wide variation in nurse practitioner certification programs and levels of testing. There was also uneven enforcement of admission requirements for certification. The NCSBN has continued to emphasize that all

Advanced Practice Registered Nurse certification organizations must develop "...legally defensible, psychometrically sound nurse practitioner examinations" that state boards of nursing could rely on in granting state authorization to nurse practitioners.[27]

STANDARDIZATION OF WOMEN'S HEALTH NURSE PRACTITIONER EDUCATION

By the early to mid 1990s more and more nurse practitioner programs were preparing WHNPs at the master's level, although there was still no requirement for a master's degree to take the NCC certification examination or by state boards of nursing for recognition as a WHNP. The standard of a master's degree to practice was becoming more urgent for WHNPs due to increased difficulty with third-party reimbursement, increased confusion of the public and health care professionals over educational requirements, the expansion of the role requiring more in-depth knowledge of women's health beyond just family planning and prenatal care, and more states requiring a higher degree for nurse practitioner licensure.[28] In 1997 the Expert Panel on Women's Health of the American Academy of Nursing (AAN) recommended the transformation of women's health services to more effectively meet women's comprehensive health care needs. The panel's recommendations included broadening nursing education at the advanced practice level to emphasize primary care of women, developing new practice models for care, advancing policy to aid in reimbursement, fewer restrictive practice acts, and redefining women's health care.[29]

As early as 1992 the American Nurses Association (ANA) merged its Council of Clinical Nurse Specialists and the Council of Nurse Practitioners into the Council of Advanced Practice Nursing. At that time ANA defined the advanced clinical practice role as based on a graduate degree in nursing and a clear definition of the skills of the advanced practice nurse (APN).[30] In the same year, the NCSBN defined advanced practice nursing as a licensed registered nurse with a graduate degree and education in a specialized area.[27] Increasingly more state boards of nursing required a master's degree for state recognition as a nurse practitioner. With the expansion of the definition of women's health care as encompassing the entire lifespan to include prevention, maintenance, and restoration of health, it became clear that advanced education was required. With strong urging from the NCSBN, NCC made the decision to require a master's degree of nurses seeking certification for the WHNP by January 1, 2007; thereby establishing the master's as the entry level.[13] Certificate nurse practitioner programs are no longer recognized, and only a master's degree or a post-master's certificate in women's health is accepted as the educational standard to sit for the certification examination in women's health and by state boards of nursing for licensure or authority to practice.[27,29] As the educational requirements of the WHNP became better defined, the role was expanding into the primary care realm as part of the NONPF competencies and curriculum guidelines, and as a component of the certification examination by NCC.

DEVELOPMENT OF A MORE INCLUSIVE MODEL OF WOMEN'S HEALTH

In the 1990s there was a move within medicine to establish a specialty in women's health. Nursing, on the other hand, has made women's health an integral part of nursing curricula (undergraduate and graduate), and the health care system through practice and research for many years. However, nursing continues to fragment the care given to women by training nurses and APNs to manage only certain portions of a woman's lifespan (i.e. prenatal, reproductive years, childhood). Walker and Tinkle[31] highlighted this fragmentation and made a case for moving toward an integrative science of women's health. Integrative science is a means of viewing the woman holistically and "…bringing together phenomena relevant to women." Because childbearing is viewed as a discrete portion of a woman's life the relationship of that pregnancy to her overall health promotion, maintenance, and management of chronic health problems before and after that pregnancy can be overlooked. Fragmentation of health care for women is perpetuated by the health care delivery system. According to Walker and Tinkle, the lack of ongoing comprehensive management and absence of linkages between pregnancy care and women's ongoing health care create disconnects between issues that arise during pregnancy and the future health of women. Weight gain during pregnancy with its long-term implications for cardiovascular health and the likelihood of the onset of type II diabetes following gestational diabetes mellitus are examples of this fragmentation.

Women's health nurse practitioners are in a key position to provide such care to women across the lifespan. But the knowledge base must be expanded to allow this extension of services. With the entry level of education for the WHNP currently at the master's level and the doctorate of nursing practice in the near future, nursing has the opportunity to fill the void in women's health care through practice, research, education, and collaboration with other health care providers.

PRIMARY CARE VERSUS SPECIALTY CARE IN WOMEN'S HEALTH

In 1995 the Pew Foundation published a recommendation for health professional training of physicians, nurses, and pharmacists. The suggestion was that all students in health professions take the same basic courses and then branch off to focus in a particular area.[32] There has been similar discussion about the education of all nurse practitioners as family nurse practitioners (FNPs) or adult nurse practitioners (ANPs) by the NCSBN. This basic generalist training would provide consistency across the advanced practice specialties and allow for further training in a specialized area, such as pediatrics or women's health. On completion of the basic education requirements, graduates would take a basic certification examination qualifying them for generalist practice or for specialization in a particular area. With the broadened focus of primary care in the WHNP role, it seems imperative that the generalist background of either an FNP or ANP as a basis for women's health specialization would provide the skills necessary to manage women's health care across the lifespan.

Women's health nurse practitioners currently lack the education and practice experience to manage multiple, complex chronic disease states in women both in middle age and in the elder years. With the baby boom generation aging rapidly, expanded education in elder care, chronic disease, medication alterations with aging, and issues specific to that age group is imperative. This broad background of education with additional focused training in women's health may seem to be becoming even more specialized, but this approach will broaden the scope of practice and make the WHNP a more marketable role. The expansion into primary care will prepare WHNPs to practice where currently they are unable, such as rural and frontier areas of the United States. This will increase women's access to health care, health promotion services, preventive care, and management of acute and chronic disease, providing for integrative health care throughout the lifespan.

SUMMARY

The role of the WHNP began as a very focused specialty in family planning. Over the past nearly 40 years the demands of the health care system and women themselves have broadened the scope of practice to include the reproductive cycle and gynecologic aspects of women's health. Nursing and WHNPs must look to an integrative science of women's health for the next step in the development of the role to include primary care across the lifespan of women, based on the generalist knowledge of the FNP/ANP and the specialist preparation of the WHNP.

REFERENCES

1. HRSA. The registered nurse population: findings from the March 2004 national sample survey of registered nurses. 2006; Available at: http://bhpr.hrsa.gov/healthworkforce/msurvey04/3.htm. Accessed March 27, 2009.
2. Kendig S. Women's health nurse practitioner. Available at: http://www.nursesource.org/womens.html. Accessed March 8, 2009.
3. About NCC. 2009; Available at: http://www.nccwebsite.org/about-ncc.aspx. Accessed February 24, 2009.
4. Taylor D, Woods N. What we know and how we know it: contributions from nursing to women's health research and scholarship. Annu Rev Nurs Res 2001;19:3–28.
5. Weisman CS. Advocating for gender-specific health care: a historical perspective. J Gend Specif Med 2000;3(3):22–4.
6. Engelhart A. Our bodies, ourselves and the women's health movement. Harv Libr Bull 2000;11(3–4):29–33.
7. Bibb BN. The effectiveness of non-physicians as providers of family planning services. JOGN Nurs 1979;8(3):137–43.
8. National Family Planning and Reproductive Health Association (NFPRH). Family planning facts: history of Title X. Available at: http://www.nfprha.org/main/family_planning.cfm?Category=History_of_Title_X&Section=Main. Accessed March 8, 2009.
9. Critchlow D. Birth control, population control, and family planning: an overview. J Policy Hist 1995;7(1):1–21.
10. Nichols FH. History of the women's health movement in the 20th century. JOGN Nurs 2000;29(1):56–64.
11. Gold RB. Title X: three decades of accomplishment. The Guttmacher Report on Public Policy. February 2001.
12. Manisoff M, Davis LW. Family planning nurse practitioners in the United States. Fam Plann Perspect 1975;7(4):154–7.
13. Lewis JS. Advanced practice in maternal/child nursing: history, current status, and thoughts about the future. MCN Am J Matern Child Nurs 2000;25(6):327–30.
14. Burchell RC. Extended role of the nurse practitioner in obstetric and gynecologic practice at Hartford Hospital. JOGN Nurs 1972;1(4):52–3.
15. Willson J. Health care for women: present deficiencies and future needs. Obstet Gynecol 1970;36:178–86.
16. MacBride O. An overview of the health professions educational assistance act, 1963-1971. New Brunswick (NJ): Robert Wood Johnson Foundation; June 1973.
17. The culture of family planning: an HCET learninglink on-line training module. 2009; Available at: http://wwwhcet.org/training/FPculture.htm#intro. Accessed March 8, 2009.
18. Office of Public Health and Science. Announcement of anticipated availability of funds for family planning clinical specialty training projects. Fed Regist 1999;64(55):14079–83.
19. Announcement of anticipated availability of funds for family planning clinical specialty training projects. Fed Regist 2002;67(128):44743–7.

20. Nurses Association of the American College of Obstetricians and Gynecologists (NAACOG). NAACOG statement on the role of the OB-GYN nurse practitioner. J Obstet Gynecol Neonatal Nurs 1972;1(1):56–7.
21. Association of Women's Health. Obstetric and neonatal nurses' health for women and newborns program. Nurs Outlook 1999;47(1):37–8.
22. National Organization of Nurse Practitioner Faculties (NONPF). The National Organization of Nurse Practitioner faculties: overview. 2005; Available at: http://www.nonpf.org/NONPF2005/Overview/Overview.htm. Accessed March 22, 2009.
23. National Organization of Nurse Practitioner Faculties. Advanced nursing practice: nurse practitioner curriculum guidelines. Washington, DC: NONPF; 1990.
24. National Organization of Nurse Practitioner Faculties. Advanced nursing practice: nurse practitioner curriculum guidelines. Washington, DC: HRSA; 1995.
25. National Association of Nurse Practitioners in Women's Health. NPWH Mission. 2009; Available at: http://www.npwh.org/i4a/pages/index.cfm?pageid=3333. Accessed February 28, 2009.
26. Association of Women's Health, Obstetric and Neonatal Nurses. Obstetric and Neonatal Nurses and National Association of Nurse Practitioners in Women's Health. The women's health nurse practitioner: guidelines for practice and education. Washington, DC: Association of Women's Health; 2000.
27. National Council of State Boards of Nursing (NCSBN). History of APRN. 2009; Available at: http://www.ncsbn.org/428.htm#Background_of_the_Issue. Accessed March 22, 2009.
28. Curran L. The women's health nurse practitioner: evolution of a powerful role. AWHONN Lifelines 2002;6(4):332–7.
29. American Academy of Nursing (AAN). Women's health and women's health care: recommendations of the 1996 AAN expert panel on women's health. Nurs Outlook 1997;45(1):7–15.
30. American Nurses Association Congress on Nursing Practice. Working definition: nurses in advanced clinical practice. Washington, DC: ANACNP; 1992.
31. Walker L, Tinkle M. Toward an integrative science of women's health. JOGN Nurs 1996;25(5):379–82.
32. Pew Health Professions Commission. Critical challenges: revitalizing the health professions for the twenty-first century: the third report of the Pew Health Professions Commission. San Francisco, California, December 1995.

Promoting Wellness in Women Across the Life Span

Robynn Zender, MS*, Ellen Olshansky, DNSc, WHNP-BC, FAAN

KEYWORDS

• Wellness • Women's health • Lifespan • Health promotion

Although wellness is an everyday term in the lexicon of society, scientific, and popular literature, it is often ill-defined or left to assumptions whereby perceptions of the definition differ from person to person.[1] As early as 495 to 429 BC, the feeling of well-being was linked with the presence of health by Pericles, a Greek statesman. Holistic thought was seen in Plato's era, when health care providers were encouraged to care for the whole person, as seen in his statement, "The part can never be well unless the whole is well."[1] In 1946, the World Health Organization promoted a definition of health that extended beyond simply the absence of disease, to include one's state of mental, physical, and social well-being.[1] Wikipedia reports a wellness definition from an alternative medicine perspective that expands the aforementioned aspects of health to include spiritual well-being, and the effect that balance in these dimensions has in promoting and maintaining wellness. This spiritual wellness parallels Maslow's hierarchy of self-actualization, whereby greater self-actualization reduces one's dependence on social, economic, and physical boundaries for life satisfaction, and new perspectives involving faith positively affirm life.[1] For purposes of this article, wellness is defined as an individual's subjective experience of overall life satisfaction in relation to physical, mental, emotional, spiritual, social, economic, occupational, and environmental dimensions.

Women's wellness focuses on those aspects of well-being that pertain disproportionately, or solely, to women. Wellness includes but is not limited to physical, emotional, and social aspects, and disruptions that alter a woman's quality of life, such as reproductive and hormonal issues, bone health, gastrointestinal (GI) stress, and urinary incontinence. This article discusses women's wellness through the life span, from preconception through death, and considers the implications of these issues for the nursing profession.

PRECONCEPTION

A woman's health begins long before birth, and even before conception, with the genetic and lifestyle makeups of the generations preceding her. Setting aside the topic

Program in Nursing Science, College of Health Sciences, University of California, 233 Irvine Hall, Irvine, CA 92697, USA
* Corresponding author.
E-mail address: rzender@uci.edu (R. Zender).

Nurs Clin N Am 44 (2009) 281–291
doi:10.1016/j.cnur.2009.06.009
0029-6465/09/$ – see front matter © 2009 Elsevier Inc. All rights reserved.

of heritable genetic disorders, the behaviors of a baby's mother before she becomes pregnant influence the outcome of the pregnancy more than prenatal care, a fact relatively unknown to the general public, including health care professionals.[2] Prenatal care has not demonstrated an impact on the incidence of prematurity and congenital anomalies, the leading causes of infant mortality in the United States, suggesting that prenatal care has simply begun too late.[2,3]

Most congenital anomalies can be traced to the first 17 to 56 days post conception. This time span is referred to as the organogenesis period; a critical time initiated 3 days after the first missed menstrual period. Exposures in this time frame that can impact organogenesis include maternal nutritional status (eg, folate levels), prescription and nonprescription drug use (such as isotretinoin, antiepileptics, and large doses of vitamin A), tobacco and alcohol use, underlying maternal diseases (such as diabetes), and environmental exposures, all of which could be addressed in a preconceptional education program. Other poor pregnancy outcomes, such as low birth weight, placental abruption, ectopic pregnancy, and placenta previa, might also be prevented by preconception counseling (eg, on smoking cessation).[2]

Along a similar vein internatal care, a package of health care and ancillary services provided to a woman and her family from the birth of one child to the birth of her next child, offers an opportunity for wellness promotion between pregnancies.[3] Internatal care has the potential for maximum effectiveness with high-risk mothers, such as women living with chronic conditions (eg, hypertension, diabetes, or weight problems) or prior adverse pregnancy outcomes like prematurity and fetal death, which carry high recurrence risk in subsequent pregnancies.[3] Biobehavioral risk factors are also often carried from one pregnancy into the next.[3]

Because proposed topics for preconception and internatal care are numerous and debatable, a workgroup and subsequent select panel was formed in 2005 through the Centers for Disease Control and Prevention.[4] The members of this group provided the strongest recommendations for the following clinical intervention topics to be made available to all women and their partners as part of routine primary care, irrespective of desire for pregnancy: family planning, weight status, nutrient intake (calcium, iron, and iodine), folate, immunizations, substance use (alcohol and tobacco), sexually transmitted infections, hepatitis B, measles/mumps/rubella, human immunodeficiency virus, *Chlamydia*, syphilis, diabetes mellitus, thyroid disease, phenylketonuria, seizure disorders, hypertension, rheumatoid arthritis, household exposures (undefined), prescription and over-the-counter medications, use of herbal supplements, weight loss products, and sport supplements, reproductive history (prior preterm birth, prior cesarean delivery, and prior miscarriage), and women with cancer (newly diagnosed and cancer survivors).[4,5]

INFANCY

There are many interventions important to promoting wellness in infancy. In newborns, delayed cord clamping, Apgar scoring, vitamin K injections, eye drops, and phenylketonuria screening are routine procedures and, in infants, health screenings, immunizations, and sudden infant death syndrome and shaken baby syndrome education may be part of health promotion. These interventions improve outcomes for all babies, not merely girl babies, and so this article discusses two wellness-promoting activities that may have implications for women in particular: breastfeeding and vitamin D supplementation.

The benefits of breastfeeding to infants regardless of gender are well documented, including a lower risk of sudden death syndrome;[6] suffering fewer infectious illnesses;

scoring higher on cognitive, IQ, and visual acuity tests at school age; a lower risk of some cancers (Hodgkin disease and childhood leukemia); a lower risk for juvenile-onset diabetes; significant protection against asthma and eczema; possibly a lower risk for obesity in childhood and adolescence; and having fewer cavities and being less likely to require braces.[7] Indirect benefits of breastfeeding to infants include the benefits to breastfeeding mothers, such as a reduced risk of ovarian and premenopausal breast cancers, osteoporosis, long-term obesity, and anemia, enjoying greater confidence and less anxiety than bottle-feeding mothers, a quicker recovery from childbirth, and having stronger feelings of attachment between a mother and her child.[7]

However, breastfeeding may also benefit girl babies disproportionately, both in childhood and later life, by reducing the risk of inflammatory bowel disease, which includes two major disorders: Crohn disease and ulcerative colitis.[7–9] Crohn disease presents in women at a slightly higher rate than in men, whereas ulcerative colitis has a slightly higher prevalence in men.[7–9] Breastfeeding has been shown to have a greater protective effect for Crohn disease than for ulcerative colitis.[9]

In a 2007 survey by the Centers for Disease Control (CDC) of all United States hospitals and birth centers, maternity care in birth facilities in most states were found not to be fully supportive of breastfeeding, a phenomenon found in particular in the southern region of the United States, where the lowest rates of breastfeeding and maternity practice scores exist. The US Breastfeeding Committee recommends exclusive breastfeeding for the first 6 months of life, with gradual introduction of solid foods after 6 months.[7]

Vitamin D is a critical nutrient for bone health at all stages in life because it is essential for the absorption of dietary calcium and phosphorus.[10] A vitamin D deficiency in utero and during childhood can lead to growth retardation, altered brain development, and skeletal deformities, and may increase the risk of chronic disease (such as type 1 diabetes and altered mental function), hip fracture, and osteoporosis later in life.[10–12] Osteoporosis is found in women at eight times more than in men, according to the National Osteoporosis Foundation, although it occurs in all populations at all ages.[11] Osteoporosis was originally characterized as a pediatric disorder that manifested itself in old age, with its roots starting in fetal life.[11] Maternal circulating vitamin D concentrations during the third trimester of pregnancy have been correlated with skeletal size of the offspring at birth and 1 year, and with prepubertal bone mineral density at 9 years.[11]

Adequate calcium and vitamin D intake is crucial to achieving peak bone mass for the preservation of bone mass throughout life.[11] The most important factor affecting serum vitamin D levels is exposure to the sun, whereby it is converted in the skin and, subsequently, in the liver and kidney into usable vitamin D.[10,11] Human breast milk contains little vitamin D and women who are vitamin D deficient provide even less of this nutrient to their breast-fed infant.[10,13] It is therefore recommended that breast-fed infants receive 400 IU of vitamin D_3 per day, with 1000 to 2000 IU of vitamin D_3 per day being safe, or measured sun exposure.[10,13] It is recommended that lactating mothers receive 1000 to 2000 IU of vitamin D_3 per day, with up to 4000 IU per day being safe when sustained for 5 months.[10,13]

YOUTH AND ADOLESCENCE

One of the most important determinants of bone health in later life is peak bone mass (the achievement of the full genetic potential for bone density), which is accrued largely during puberty.[11,12,14] A recent study found the population with the lowest circulating vitamin D concentrations to be adolescents.[15] Action to maximize peak bone mass should be taken during the childhood years to ensure young girls and their caregivers receive information on preventing osteoporosis and related fractures later in life. Lypaczewski and colleagues developed a creative and fun educational program to achieve exactly this, and they tested it through a Girl Scouts program in Omaha, Nebraska, with 9-year-old girls. The program can serve as a template for bone health education in girls between the ages of 9 and 12 years.[14]

A second area of wellness care in young girls relates to the rising incidence of precocious puberty: the appearance of secondary sex characteristics before the age of 8 years, or the onset of menarche before age 9.[16] Girls with precocious puberty present the appearance of mature physiologic readiness for sexuality and childbearing while retaining immature psychosocial characteristics, signaling a lack of preparedness for intimate relationships and decision making.[16] Precocious puberty has a prevalence of 1 in 5000 children and exists more in girls than boys at a ratio of 10:1.[16] Studies indicate that girls who become sexually mature at earlier ages are more likely to engage in risk-taking behaviors such as smoking, using alcohol or drugs, and engaging in unprotected sex.[16]

Risk factors for precocious puberty include non-Hispanic Black ethnicity (although it is evident in Caucasian and Hispanic girls), obesity, genetic predisposition, maternal malnutrition during pregnancy, small for gestational age at birth, environmental exposures to endocrine disruptive toxins (such as pesticides, polychlorinated biphenyls, soy products, plastics, food preservatives, some beauty products, exogenous sex steroids used in assisted reproductive technology, and some prescription medications), and psychosocial stress (low socioeconomic status, peer pressure, violence, bullying, performance pressure, and sexual abuse).[16] Recommendations for nursing education of parents with at-risk children include avoiding childhood exposures to pesticides, herbicides, and insecticides; washing fruits and vegetables before consumption; buying plastic toys or other products (shower curtains, for example) labeled "non-PVC" or "nonphthalate"; avoiding plastics bearing the number "3"; teaching good hand-washing practices; not microwaving food in plastic containers; drinking filtered water; and controlling weight through diet and exercise.[16]

Adolescents and young women have unique health needs relating to the risks and consequences for contracting infections, date rape, drug and alcohol use and abuse, the development of eating disorders, distorted body image, and unhealthy means of controlling one's weight. Emotionality (in particular, anger), sleep disturbances, and urinary incontinence also present uniquely in adolescents, and knowledge of and sensitivity to these topics by the nursing professional can provide essential support to this population.[17–20]

ADULT
Premenstrual Syndrome

Premenstrual syndrome (PMS) is characterized by the cyclic recurrence of physical, psychological, and behavioral symptoms during the luteal phase of the menstrual cycle, and can have a severe debilitating effect on the quality of life for some women.[21–23] Premenstrual dysphoric disorder (PMDD) is considered the most severe presentation of PMS, and presents with at least one mood symptom (typically low mood, tension, anger, irritability, or mood swings) and suffering physical or psychological symptoms in most menstrual cycles in the past year.[22,23] As many as 80% of reproductive-aged women experience at least a few symptoms of physical discomfort or mood changes premenstrually, but clinical prevalences are estimated at between 19% and 30% for PMS, and 3% and 8% for PMDD.[23] The etiology of PMS is unknown.

Clinical significance of both disorders, by definition, affect quality of life in one or more areas of interpersonal relationships, social behavior, work attendance, or work productivity, and rate comparably on health-related quality-of-life scores with dysthymic disorders, and not much better than those of major depressive disorder.[23] PMDD-affected women also score lower on quality-of-life measures than those with back pain, and about equally with type 2 diabetes, hypertension, osteoarthritis and rheumatoid arthritis sufferers, and women with depression, which illustrates the dramatic impact of this disorder.[23]

Current treatment relies on self-management, dietary modifications, exercise, stress management, cognitive-behavioral therapies, and fortified coping strategies.[21,22] Some prescription and nonprescription medications have been used, as well as a variety of complementary medicine (energetic touch therapies, craniosacral manipulation, art and music therapy, and ceremonial events)[21] and alternative medicine (acupuncture, herbal medicine, massage, hypnosis)[24] therapies.[21,22]

Vitamin D Deficiency

As in infancy, childhood, and adolescence, vitamin D status has important implications for the health of women in their adult years. A decline in serum vitamin D status has occurred over the past 10 to 15 years,[11] with an estimated 1 billion people worldwide, and between 40% to 100% of United States and European elderly men and women still living in the community (not in nursing homes) having vitamin D deficiency.[10,25] Circulating concentrations of vitamin D are affected by body weight (having an inverse relationship), use of sun protection, and milk intake.[15] Undiagnosed vitamin D deficiency is not uncommon.[10,25]

In addition to skeletal effects, vitamin D deficiency has been linked to an increased risk for other diseases, both acute and chronic, including influenza,[10,11] tuberculosis,[10,11] diabetes,[10,11] rheumatoid arthritis,[10,11] certain cancers (colon, prostate, and breast),[10,11] hypertension,[10] congestive heart failure,[10] schizophrenia,[10] depression,[10] and multiple sclerosis (MS), a disease that affects women two to three times more than men, according to the National MS Society.[10,11] With adequate sun exposure, supplementation for vitamin D is unnecessary.[10] Depending on time of day, season, latitude, and skin pigmentation, exposure of arms and legs for 5 to 30 minutes between the hours of 10 AM and 3 PM twice a week is often adequate.[10] A circulating concentration of 30 ng per milliliter (70–80 nmol/L) of 25-hydroxyvitamin D or more (intoxication is possible, but rare) is thought to be optimal.[10,11,25]

Irritable Bowel Syndrome

Irritable bowel syndrome (IBS) is one of the most common gastrointestinal disorders in adult primary care, gastroenterology, and psychiatric settings, affecting an estimated 20% of the United States population, and causing significant impairment in quality of life for those afflicted.[26–30] IBS is often diagnosed by exclusion of organic disease,[26,27,31] and is characterized by abdominal bloating, abdominal discomfort or pain, and a change in bowel habits.[26,27] IBS is seen in far greater numbers in women than men.[26,29,30]

Although IBS has no known etiology and no biomarker for diagnosis, a recent study implicates a gender-dependent immune mechanism in a subset of IBS sufferers.[32] Aside from this, IBS is more generally thought of within a biopsychosocial model, in which physiologic symptoms such as altered gut motility and increased visceral sensitivity are linked to psychological, environmental, and social factors such as life stressors, psychological stress, coping skills, and personality.[31] IBS impacts both physical and emotional aspects of a patient's life with anxiety reactions, a sense of helplessness resulting from uncontrollable symptoms, embarrassment, and guilt from canceling social engagements and burdening family members. Physical effects of the illness include fatigue (extreme exhaustion) and pain, as well as restricting diet and activities for the unpredictable nature of the illness.[29] IBS has varying, individualistic, and often confusing presentations that make diagnosing, understanding, and treating the disorder challenging.[27–29]

Treatment for IBS is often administered on a trial-and-error basis using several medications or cognitive-behavioral therapy,[29] as well as complementary and alternative medicine strategies, stress management, patient education, and dietary changes.[28] Other coping mechanisms found to be used frequently and as a significant part of a woman's day-to-day routine include possessing a positive attitude, support from family and friends, controlling surroundings and situations, and distraction or ignoring the problem.[28] Frontline nurses have the opportunity to improve the quality of life for those suffering from IBS through understanding the individual symptoms any one patient is experiencing through health and diet diaries, detailed health histories, and goal setting. General education of IBS, as well as targeted education to minimize the cascade of effects that occur from the onset of an IBS attack, referrals to dietitians, and a focus on self-empowerment and active participation in self-management all play a role in managing lifelong gastrointestinal disorders such as IBS.[28,29]

Sleep Disorders

Insomnia and restless leg syndrome have a significant impact on overall health and quality of life, and are generally treatable.[33] Insomnia differs from short-term sleep disturbance in that insomnia is a chronic and frequently reported difficulty with sleep induction or maintenance or nonrestorative sleep, lasting a minimum of 1 month, and is associated with significant impairment in social, occupational, or other areas of functioning.[33] Insomnia is associated with significant morbidity including reduced quality of life, falls in the elderly, increased absenteeism, and risk of developing major depression, and affects women in greater numbers than men, a trend which increases with age.[33] The risk for developing insomnia does not emerge until puberty, suggesting a possible contribution of hormonal changes.[33] The prevalence of insomnia is estimated at between 9% and 15% in the general population.[33]

Comorbid conditions occur commonly with insomnia, including major depression, dysthymia, and chronic pain disorders, although determining direction of causality, if any exists, is difficult.[33] Treatment typically includes behavioral (cognitive therapy) and pharmacologic approaches, with success seen for both.[33]

Restless leg syndrome (RLS) is characterized by an urge to move the legs or other limbs during periods of rest or inactivity, and may affect as much as 10% of the population, with consistently higher rates seen in women.[33] Risk factors include anemia, end-stage renal disease, and pregnancy, all conditions that have iron deficiency in common.[33] Adults with symptoms of RLS may be at higher risk for sleep apnea, insomnia, anxiety, depression, drowsy driving, being late for work, absenteeism, and making errors at work.[33] Treatment often includes behavioral and pharmacologic (dopaminergic compounds) approaches, with exercise often providing some benefit. Folic acid for pregnant women, and iron replacement, as well as anecdotal accounts of relief with massage, caffeine and alcohol abstinence, vitamins, and hot baths have been reported.[33] Women are more likely to have sleep complaints than are men for several reasons, including hormonal changes throughout the life span, and increased awareness of their presentation and impact on a woman's health by nursing practitioners can greatly improve the quality of life for these patients.

Chronic Disease

Chronic disease is referred to as the health care challenge of this century.[34] It is projected that by the year 2050, nearly half of the United States population will be living with at least one chronic disease.[34] Scientific developments (ie, immunizations, antibiotics, sterilization) in the late nineteenth and early twentieth centuries led to an increased reliance on the expert advice of doctors and reduced active participation in health by individuals, but the current shift in predominant disease patterns from acute to chronic requires a move toward long-term management of chronic diseases with a focus on self-care for the individual to manage one's own health.[34]

Self-care, a person's taking responsibility for his or her own health and well-being through staying fit and healthy in all dimensions (physically, mentally, socially, and perhaps spiritually), including taking action to prevent illness and accidents, and appropriately administering medicines and treatment for minor ailments, is the underlying concept for the shift toward chronic disease management.[34] Power dynamics have been discussed as a significant factor limiting the implementation of self-care programs, with health professionals retaining the belief that they are the experts and must mediate information control.[34] It has been posited that the biggest stumbling block to successful self-care is a health professional's fear of empowering the patient.[34] Therefore for nurses, understanding the underlying paradigm from which they practice, knowing their own self-care needs, and choosing a reflective style of practice can illuminate hidden assumptions and shift the nurse's role from that of teacher or gatekeeper to one of facilitator and partner in health education and promotion.[34] Underlying this philosophy is a conceptual shift from "feeling responsible *for* patients to feeling responsible *to* patients."[34]

MENOPAUSE, OLD AGE, AND END OF LIFE
Menopause

Postmenopausal health is a growing area of medicine as the population's age and life expectancy increases, and given that women live longer than men.[35] In 2002, 7% of the total population were older than 65 years. This figure is projected to increase to 17% by the year 2050, with most elderly people living in the developed world, and few in Africa and the Near East.[35] Managing the health of menopausal and postmenopausal women from the standpoint of ovarian failure as well as aging, because estrogen deficiency affects many organ systems, mandates a holistic approach.[35]

Although the process of menopause is a natural one, many women experience at least some of the symptoms of menopause, and the risks for cardiovascular disease, osteoporotic fracture, dementia, depression, and anxiety increase after menopause, forcing the consideration of medical management of this transition.[35,36] Treatment options include hormone replacement therapy (HRT) (a source of great controversy), antidepressant and antianxiety medications, alternative medicine (such as extracted botanicals like black cohosh and evening primrose, relaxation techniques, yoga, tai chi, acupuncture, and biofeedback), and lifestyle changes in diet, exercise, and the consumption of alcohol and tobacco.[36]

Amid discussions with menopausal women regarding medical treatment of symptoms, it is important to be ever mindful of the normalcy of the menopausal process, as noted by the experiences of women with previous infertility.[37] Women who experienced infertility during their reproductive years and developed an identity of being abnormal were able to reconcile feeling different and separate during the menopause, and now felt a camaraderie with women as a group and able to participate in larger women's issues.[37] By having a complete personal history and knowledge about health issues related to aging and menopause, including menopausal symptoms and treatments, nurses skilled in counseling techniques can provide clear, accurate written information, and assist in the clarification of personal values and goals in light of medical information, ultimately helping women make appropriate decisions given their individual situation.[36,37]

Vitamin D Deficiency and Osteoporosis

Approximately 33% of women aged 60 to 70 and 60% of those 80 years or older have osteoporosis, and an estimated 47% of women and 22% of men 50 years or older will sustain an osteoporotic fracture in their remaining lifetime.[10] Studies report that elderly women given 1200 mg calcium and 800 IU of vitamin D_3 enjoy the greatest benefit in terms of prevention of hip and other nonvertebral fractures, and that 1000 mg of calcium supplementation in conjunction with 400 IU of vitamin D_3 (the current recommended dose) resulted in an increased risk of kidney stones with no reduction in risk of hip fractures.[10] Maximum benefit of calcium use appears to occur at about 30 ng per milliliter (70–80 nmol/L) serum concentration of 25(OH)D, which can be achieved and maintained only if doses higher than the current recommendation are taken.[10,25]

Living with a Disability

As the global population ages, particularly those in developed nations, an increased number of older people living with a disability can be expected because the incidence of disability increases with age.[38] In 2001, a study found that 23% of people older than 65 years were living with a disability, with the rate increasing to 65% in those older than 80 years.[38] Quality of life for older people living with a disability depends on a complex mix of base factors, including health, social connectedness, sense of self, and financial security, which are influenced by other forces such as individual adaptive responses (psychological resources such as mental outlook, attitudes, and personality characteristics) and living environment.[38] As health functioning worsens, many disabled patients redefine health in terms of abilities rather than an absence of illness.[38,39] Supportive care from nurses for the elderly living with a disability should focus attention on a person's abilities to develop the internal resources of individuals. Having free access to pertinent information, advocating for resources, and ensuring that services are responsive to an individual's needs also help to facilitate coping and adaptation through empowerment.[38]

DEATH AND DYING

People with injuries and disabilities have the expectation of a return to health, whereas those who are dying find that the process of becoming whole again means adapting to a new way of living in a world where health and wellness are celebrated, and death and dying are hidden.[40] Death is part of nature's ongoing cycle, but the nature of the disease determines how a person will die. Because of the uniqueness of every individual death and because death has become something not to be discussed, the process of dying has moved away from the home and has become medicalized, and thus dependent on professionals and institutions.[40]

How people cope with dying can be determined by the things that give meaning to their lives: the preservation of dignity, a sense of control, good pain and symptom management, having ample opportunity to integrate one's prognosis, aesthetics of the environment, ability to continue to manage one's life and relationships and understand the changes that are occurring, the importance of friends' roles in informal care, to be seen as a whole person beyond the illness, to give permission for the living to move on with their lives, and for women to continue caregiving despite serious illness.[40] In the search for an explanation of what is wrong with them, people tell their story. As this story evolves and becomes spoken it takes on a life of its own, revealing an individual's understanding and perception of her own illness and how her illness is addressed by others. Professionals sometimes need to abandon the role of expert and allow families to educate them about their experiences. In this way, dying becomes a mutually reciprocal process.[40]

Recent research supports the abandonment of making generalizations about the way people confront dying from a presupposed model of coping, to adopting of a model in which individual differences are recognized.[40] By telling her story as it is experienced, the dying individual can direct one's own life and well-being by applying influence on getting her needs met. The ways in which a patient's body is affected by the disease process and the medical treatments given determine how they live their lives, and how health care professionals, family, and friends regard the dying person has a great influence on the experience of dying.[40]

SUMMARY

Wellness is an individual's subjective experience of overall life satisfaction in relation to physical, mental, emotional, social, economic, occupational, and environmental dimensions. In keeping with the multifaceted nature of wellness, health care professionals must approach each individual from a holistic frame of reference, and have a clear understanding of her own self-care needs to serve effectively in the shifting dynamics of health and disease. Wellness care for women is unique, given their hormonal profiles, tendency to present with certain diseases disproportionately to men, and greater longevity. From preconception through death, nurses can improve the quality of life for women through acquiring knowledge, and providing education and counseling on the myriad of issues that affect well-being for each situation or diagnosis at each stage in life.

REFERENCES

1. Kiefer RA. An integrative review of the concept of well-being. Holist Nurs Pract 2008;22(5):244–52.
2. Moos MK. Preconceptional health promotion: progress in changing a prevention paradigm. J Perinat Neonatal Nurs 2004;18(1):2–13.
3. Lu MC, Kotelchuck M, Culhane JF, et al. Preconception care between pregnancies: the content of internatal care. Matern Child Health J 2006;10:S107–22.
4. Jack BW, Atrash H, Coonrod DV, et al. The clinical content of preconception care: an overview and preparation of this supplement. Am J Obstet Gynecol 2008; 199(6 Suppl 2):S266–79.
5. Moos MK, Dunlop AL, Jack BW, et al. Healthier women, healthier reproductive outcomes: recommendations for the routine care of all women of reproductive age. Am J Obstet Gynecol 2008;199(6 Suppl 2):S280–9.
6. Vennemann MM, Bajanowski T, Brinkmann B, et al. Does breastfeeding reduce the risk of sudden infant death syndrome? Pediatrics 2009;123(3):e406–10.
7. United States Breastfeeding Committee. Benefits of breastfeeding [issue paper]. Releigh (NC): United States Breastfeeding Committee; 2002.
8. Inflammatory Bowel Disease (IBD). National Center for Chronic Disease Prevention and Health Promotion. Sep 2007. Available at: http://www.cdc.gov/nccdphp/dach/ibd.htm.

9. Mikhailov TA, Furner SE. Breastfeeding and genetic factors in the etiology of inflammatory bowel disease in children. World J Gastroenterol 2009;15(3):270–9.

10. Holick MF. Vitamin D deficiency. N Engl J Med 2007;357:266–81.

11. Kimball S, Fuleihan G, Vieth R. Vitamin D: a growing perspective. Crit Rev Clin Lab Sci 2008;45(4):339–414.

12. Calcium and Bone Health. Division of Nutrition, Physical Activity and Obesity. National Center for Chronic Disease Prevention and Health Promotion. Dec 2008. Available at: http://www.cdc.gov/nutrition/everyone/basics/vitamins/calcium.html.

13. Taylor SN, Wagner CL, Hollis BW. Vitamin D supplementation during lactation to support infant and mother. J Am Coll Nutr 2008;27(6):690–701.

14. Lypaczewski F, Lappe J, Stubby J. Mom and me and healthy bones: an innovative approach to teaching bone health. Orthop Nurs 2002;21(2):35–42.

15. Looker AC, Pfeiffer CM, Lacher DA, et al. Serum 25-hydroxy vitamin D status of the US Population: 1988–1994 compared with 2000–2004. Am J Clin Nutr 2008;88:1519–27.

16. Cesario SK, Hughes LA. Precocious puberty: a comprehensive review of literature. J Obstet Gynecol Neonatal Nurs 2007;36(3):263–74.

17. Graves VA. The unique health needs of young women: application for occupational health nurses. AAOHN J 2005;53(7):320–7.

18. Vallido T, Jackson D, O'Brien L. Mad, sad and hormonal: the gendered nature of adolescent sleep disturbance. J Child Health Care 2009;13(1):7–18.

19. Van Daalen-Smith C. Living as a chameleon: girls, anger, and mental health. J Sch Nurs 2008;24(3):116–23.

20. Dockter M, Becker E, Huber CL, et al. The prevalence of urinary incontinence in high school females: implications for prevention and wellness education. J Womens Health Phys Ther 2008;32(2):7–11.

21. Shin KR, Ha JU, Park JH, et al. The effect of hand acupuncture therapy and hand moxibustion therapy on premenstrual syndrome among Korean women. West J Nurs Res 2009;31(2):171–86.

22. Stearns S. PMS and PMDD in the domain of mental health nursing. J Psychosoc Nurs Ment Health Serv 2001;39(1):16–27.

23. Yang M, Wallenstein G, Hagan M, et al. Burden of premenstrual dysphoric disorder on health- related quality of life. J Womens Health (Larchmt) 2008; 17(1):113–21.

24. Kendall ML. Integrative medicine: taking the lead in holistic palliation. J Hosp Palliat Nurs 1999;1(2):56–61.

25. Lappe JM, Davies M, Travers-Gustafson D, et al. Vitamin D status in a rural postmenopausal female population. J Am Coll Nutr 2006;25(5):395–402.

26. Park HJ, Jarrett M, Cain K, et al. Psychological distress and GI symptoms are related to severity of bloating in women with irritable bowel syndrome. Res Nurs Health 2008;31:98–107.

27. Fletcher PC, Jamieson AE, Schneider MA, et al. "I know this is bad for me, but." A qualitative investigation of women with irritable bowel syndrome and inflammatory bowel disease, part II. Clin Nurse Spec 2008;22(4):184–91.

28. Fletcher PC, Schneider MA, Van Ravenswaay V, et al. "I am doing the best that I can!" Living with inflammatory bowel disease and/or irritable bowel syndrome (part II). Clin Nurse Spec 2008;22(6):278–85.

29. Schneider MA, Fletcher PC. "I feel as if my IBS is keeping me hostage!" Exploring the negative impact of irritable bowel syndrome (IBS) and inflammatory bowel disease (IBD) upon university-aged women. Int J Nurs Pract 2008;14:135–48.

30. Leserman J, Drossman DA. Relationship of abuse history to functional gastrointestinal disorders and symptoms. Trauma Violence Abuse 2007;8(3):331–43.
31. Hertig VL, Cain KC, Jarrett ME, et al. Daily stress and gastrointestinal symptoms in women with irritable bowel syndrome. Nurs Res 2007;56(6):399–406.
32. Cremon C, Gargano L, Morselli-Labate AM, et al. Mucosal immune activation in irritable bowel syndrome: gender-dependence and association with digestive symptoms. Am J Gastroenterol 2009;104:392–400.
33. Phillips BA, Collop NA, Drake C, et al. Sleep disorders and medical conditions in women. Proceedings of the women and sleep workshop, National Sleep Foundation, Washington, DC, March 5–6, 2007. J Womens Health (Larchmt) 2008;17(7): 1191–9.
34. Wilkinson A, Whitehead L. Evolution of the concept of self-care and implications for nurses: a literature review. Int J Nurs Stud 2009;46(8):1143.
35. Lumsden MA, Rees M. Menopause and menopause transition. Preface and introduction. Best Pract Res Clin Obstet Gynaecol 2009;23(1):1–6.
36. Strayer DA, Walsh K. Menopause: decision process regarding treatment options. Available at: Cinahl Information Systems. Accessed March 2, 2009.
37. Olshansky E. Feeling normal: women's experiences of menopause after infertility. MCN Am J Matern Child Nurs 2005;30(3):195–200.
38. Murphy K, Cooney A, Shea EO, et al. Determinants of quality of life for older people living with a disability in the community. J Adv Nurs 2009;65(3):606–15.
39. Gattuso S. Becoming a wise old woman: resilience and wellness in later life. Health Sociol Rev 2003;12(2):171–7.
40. McKechnie R, MacLeod R, Keeling S. Facing uncertainty: the lived experience of palliative care. Palliat Support Care 2007;5:367–76.

Human Papillomavirus and the HPV Vaccine: Are the Benefits Worth the Risks?

Mary Knudtson, DNSc, NP, FAAN[a],*, Susan Tiso, MN, NP[b], Susanne Phillips, MSN, NP[b]

KEYWORDS

• Human papillomavirus • Gardasil vaccine
• Sexually transmitted infections

OVERVIEW AND PREVALENCE OF HUMAN PAPILLOMAVIUS

Human Papillomavirus (HPV) is the most commonly sexually transmitted infection in the United States.[1] Recent national prevalence estimates demonstrate that more than half of sexually active men and women are infected with the HPV virus at some point in their lives.[2–5] Most infections with HPV are asymptomatic, transient, and resolve without treatment. In some patients HPV infection becomes persistent, resulting in genital warts, Pap test abnormalities, cervical cancer, anogenital cancer, and head and neck cancer. An estimated 6.2 million persons acquire new HPV infections each year in the United States.[3] The overall prevalence of HPV infection in the United States was 26.8% in females between 14 and 59 years, corresponding to 24.9 million females in this age range with HPV infection.[2,4] For women in the United States, HPV prevalence is age dependent, with the highest risk among younger females (during the sexual debut period) followed by a gradual decline across older age groups. Among sexually active females HPV prevalence was higher than in all females, at 39.6% for 14- to 19-year-olds, 49.3% for 20- to 24-year-olds, 27.8% for 25- to 29-year-olds, 27.3% for 30- to 39-year-olds, 23.9% for 40- to 49-year-olds, and 20.2% for 50- to 59-year-olds.[4] In the analysis of recent studies of the prevalence of HPV in men in the United States the prevalence was between 10% and 63%.[3] In men, risk factors related to sexual behavior were associated with HPV infection, including (1) young age at first sexual intercourse, (2) a greater number of regular, lifetime, and recent sex partners, (3) a greater number of sex partners before and during marriage, (4)

[a] Program in Nursing Science, Department of Nursing, University of California, Irvine, 234 Irvine Hall, Irvine, CA 92697, USA
[b] Program in Nursing Science, Department of Nursing, University of California, Irvine, 209 Irvine Hall, Irvine, CA 92697, USA
* Corresponding author.
E-mail address: mdknudts@uci.edu (M. Knudtson).

Nurs Clin N Am 44 (2009) 293–299
doi:10.1016/j.cnur.2009.06.005   nursing.theclinics.com
0029-6465/09/$ – see front matter © 2009 Elsevier Inc. All rights reserved.

female partners having a greater lifetime number of sexual partners, and (5) high frequency of sexual intercourse.[3] Genital areas not covered by a condom may harbor HPV infection, therefore proper condom use may not provide protection.[6] Dunne and colleagues[3] found that between 7.1% and 46.2% of men had HPV detected on their scrotum or inguinal area.

TYPES OF HUMAN PAPILLOMAVIUS

There are more than 100 different types of HPV, which differ in the type of epithelium they infect. Some HPV types infect skin sites whereas others infect mucosal surfaces. There are more than 40 HPV types that can infect mucosal surfaces, such as the ano-genital epithelium, which includes the cervix, vagina, vulva, rectum, urethra, penis, and anus, and the oral pharyngeal epithelium. HPV types are divided into low-risk and high-risk subtypes. The high-risk subtypes are considered oncogenic or cancer-associated types. The low-risk types are considered nononcogenic.

The high-risk types of HPV are found in association with invasive cancers of the cervix, vulva, penis, rectum, and oropharynx. HPV 16 is the most common high-risk type and is found in approximately half of all cervical cancers.[7] HPV 18 is another common high-risk virus type and is associated with squamous cell and glandular cell cancers of the cervix. It is responsible for 10% to 12% of cervical cancers. The other high-risk HPV subtypes may be associated with cancer but they are implicated much less frequently than HPV 16 and 18.

The low-risk types of HPV can cause benign or low-grade cervical cell changes and genital warts, and are rarely found in invasive disease. HPV 6 and 11 subtypes are most commonly associated with genital warts (**Box 1** and **Table 1**).

HUMAN PAPILLOMAVIRUS TRANSMISSION

HPV is transmitted though direct skin to skin contact. The highest risk for transmission is penetrative genital contact such as vaginal or anal intercourse.[8] Other types of genital contact can lead to HPV infection, including oral to genital, hand to genital, or genital to genital contact; transmission from these routes is less common than from sexual intercourse.

The number of partners is proportionately linked to the risk of acquiring HPV infection. Having sexual relations with a new partner may be a stronger risk factor for HPV acquisition than having sexual relations with the same regular partner.[9] The risk of HPV infection is increased if a partner has had or currently has other partners.[9]

HUMAN PAPILLOMAVIRUS INFECTION

Most patients who contract HPV infection have transient and asymptomatic infections. Seventy percent of women with HPV infection become HPV negative by DNA

| Box 1 |
| Factors associated with HPV acquisition in women |
| Young age (less than 25 years old) |
| Increased number of sexual partners |
| Early age at first intercourse (16 years or younger) |
| Male partner with multiple sex partners (current or past) |

Table 1	
Types of human papillomavirus	
High Risk	Low Risk
HPV 16, 18, 31, 33, 35, 39, 45, 51, 52, 56, 58, 59, 68, 82	HPV 6, 11, 40, 42, 43, 44, 54, 61, 72, 73, 81

testing within 1 year, and 91% become DNA HPV negative within 2 years.[9] The median duration of a new HPV infection is usually 8 months. HPV 16 infections typically persist longer than other HPV types.[10] The development of an effective immune response is thought to be the mechanism for clearance of HPV infection.

Women with transient HPV infections may develop atypical squamous cells of undetermined significance or low-grade squamous intraepithelial lesions (SIL) on Pap smear testing. These cytologic abnormalities on Pap smear are caused by HPV infection and may spontaneously clear.

About 10% of women infected with HPV develop persistent infections.[10] Women with persistent high-grade SIL HPV infection are at the greatest risk of developing cervical cancer or cervical cancer precursors, including moderate or severe dysplasia or cervical intraepithelial neoplasia (CIN 2 or 3). In addition to cervical cancer, HPV is responsible for 90% of anal cancers, 40% of vulvar, vaginal, and penile cancers, and 12% of oral and pharyngeal cancers.[11]

HUMAN PAPILLOMAVIRUS PERSISTENCE

The most important risk factor associated with invasive cervical cancer is never or rarely being screened for cervical cancer with Pap smear testing. More than half of the women in the United States diagnosed with cervical cancer have never been screened with a Pap smear and 10% have not been screened within the past 5 years.[12] Immunosuppression from any cause, including HIV infection, increases the persistence of HPV infection and the risk of invasive cervical cancer.[13] Cigarette smoking has also been associated with HPV persistence and cervical cancer risk.[14] Other factors associated with an increased risk of cervical cancer include the long-term use of oral contraceptives and coinfection such as Chlamydia.[14]

In 2007, the age-adjusted incidence rate for invasive cervical cancer in the United States was 7.9 per 100,000 women (11,150 new cases).[11] Approximately 4000 women die in the United States from cervical cancer each year. All women should continue to receive regular Pap smear testing as recommended by the Centers for Disease Control, American College of Obstetricians and Gynecologists, or the American Cancer Society, regardless of whether they have received the HPV vaccine or not.

HUMAN PAPILLOMAVIRUS VACCINE

The quadrivalent HPV vaccine (Gardasil, Merck, Whitehouse Station, New Jersey) was developed to protect against most cervical cancers and genital warts.[15] It is the first cancer prevention vaccine approved by the US Food and Drug Administration (FDA). This prophylactic vaccine works by preventing infection with four HPV types, type 16 and 18 that cause 70% of cervical cancer, and HPV 6 and 11 that cause 90% of genital warts.[11] The vaccine has no therapeutic effects on HPV-related disease, which means it will not treat existing diseases or conditions caused by prior HPV infection. Studies indicate the vaccine also provides cross-protection against infection and disease due to subtypes HPV 31, 33, 45, 52 and 58, which are not included in the vaccine.[15]

The current vaccine is FDA approved in girls and women between the ages of 9 and 26 years and consists of a 3-dose series. The intramuscular vaccination is recommended to be given initially, then at 2 and 6 months post initial vaccination. The minimal interval between doses is 1 month between doses 1 and 2, and 3 months between doses 2 and 3. It is noninfectious and nononcogenic, and it does not contain thimerosal or mercury.[11]

Human Papillomavirus Vaccine Efficacy

The immunogenicity of the quadrivalent HPV vaccine has been measured by detection of IgG antibodies to the HPV major capsid protein. In all studies to date, 99.5% of vaccine recipients developed an antibody response to all four HPV types in the vaccine 1 month after completing the three-dose series.[16] In women not previously exposed to HPV infection, the clinical trials demonstrate almost 100% vaccine efficacy in preventing cervical precancers, vulvar and vaginal precancers, and genital warts caused by the four vaccine types.[17] In women already infected with a targeted HPV type, the vaccine did not prevent disease from that virus type but did protect against the other HPV types contained within the vaccine. Antibody titers were higher in young girls (age 9–15) vaccinated with the Gardasil compared with older women (age 16–26) in the efficacy trials.[17]

Efficacy studies are in progress for the vaccine in women between age 27 and 45 years and in males. The vaccine is not FDA approved or recommended in those groups at this time.

Human Papillomavirus Vaccine Safety

The HPV vaccine has been studied in more than 11,000 girls and women between the ages of 9 and 26 years.[18] The studies have found the vaccine to be safe, without causing serious side effects. The most common adverse event was injection site pain, at 84%. This reaction was common but mild. Redness and swelling at the injection site were the next most common adverse events, at 25% each.[11] There have also been reports of syncope following vaccine administration. Syncope after any vaccine is more common in adolescents than in adults receiving vaccinations. It is recommended that vaccine recipients be seated during vaccine administration and clinicians observe patients for 15 to 20 minutes post vaccine. Fever was reported in 10% of recipients within 15 days of vaccine administration and in 9% of placebo recipients.

Advisory Committee on Immunization Practices Recommendations

The Advisory Committee on Immunization Practices (ACIP) recommends the vaccine be administered to 11- to 12-year-old girls; however, it can be administered to girls as young as 9 years old. The vaccine is also recommended for girls and women between 13 and 26 years old who have not yet received or completed the vaccine series.

Ideally the vaccine should be administered before the onset of sexual activity. Girls and women who are sexually active should receive the vaccine if they were not vaccinated before sexual debut. Females who are infected with one or more HPV types should also receive the vaccine if they are between the ages of 9 and 26 years. The vaccine will not protect them against the virus types they already have but may provide protection from the virus types they have not acquired.

Contraindications to Vaccination

A severe allergic reaction to a vaccine component or following a prior dose of HPV vaccine is a contraindication to receipt of a subsequent HPV vaccine. A moderate or severe illness is a precaution to vaccination, and vaccination should be deferred until the symptoms of the acute illness have improved; however, a minor acute illness with or without fever is not a reason to defer vaccination. HPV vaccination is not recommended in pregnancy.

DISCUSSION

Cervical cancer has claimed the lives of more women in the United States than any other type of cancer.[7,18] Over the past 40 years, cervical cancer screening using the Pap smear test and treatment of precancerous cervical abnormalities has dramatically reduced the incidence of cervical cancer and mortality in the United States.[19] Although approximately 82% of women in the United States have been screened with a Pap smear test in the past 3 years, screening programs are not reaching all women. Half of the women in the United States diagnosed with cervical cancer have never been screened.[20] Studies demonstrate that cervical cancer disproportionately affects women of lower socioeconomic status, especially those without regular access to health care, who are uninsured, and who are recent immigrants.[21]

Sexually transmitted infections are common among sexually active adolescents. It is estimated that 46% of all high school students have sexual intercourse by the time they graduate from high school, and 75% of young adults have intercourse before they marry.[19] The Center for Disease Control estimates that 3.2 million adolescent girls have a sexually transmitted infection. Among sexually active females in the United States, HPV prevalence for 14- to 19-year-olds was 39.6% and for 20- to 24-year-olds 49.3%.[4]

The HPV vaccine can reduce the incidence of cervical cancer and genital warts, thereby reducing suffering and harm. Vaccine efficacy was close to 100% for the prevention of precancerous lesions for girls and women who were not exposed or infected with HPV before receiving the vaccine, and has been found to be the highest in the youngest vaccine recipients. Studies have demonstrated that antibody titers are highest in the younger age groups (9–15 years) compared with older girls (16–26 years).[22] Vaccinating girls at a younger age may provide a stronger immune response and may protect them from infection before sexual debut.

The ACIP weighs the known and potential benefits against known risks before a vaccine is recommended. During the clinical trails of the HPV vaccine and post licensure, no serious adverse events in girls or women have been reported in women who received the vaccine compared with those who received the placebo. The ACIP determined that the benefits of vaccination outweigh the risk of vaccination with the Gardasil vaccine.

Due to the high prevalence of HPV infection in sexually active adolescents and young adults, vaccination with Gardasil to prevent HPV infection is recommended. The benefits clearly outweigh the risks.

Nursing Implications

The nursing implications for the HPV vaccine are related to education and counseling of parents and patients regarding HPV vaccination, and for young adult women for whom the vaccine is indicated. It is important for nurses to understand the risk factors, prevalence, and implications of HPV infection in women to be able to counsel them appropriately. Patients and parents should be counseled on the different types of

HPV, the factors associated with HPV acquisition in women, the modes of transmission, and how to reduce their risk for infection, as well as the potential short-term and long-term consequences of persistent HPV infection.

In addition, it is important for nurses to educate parents and patients about the HPV vaccine itself. Parents and patients should be educated on the efficacy of the vaccine, the recommended schedule for vaccination, and the potential side effects of the vaccine. It is important for them to understand that this is a cancer prevention vaccine approved by the FDA and that it does not treat existing HPV infection or diseases in previously infected patients. Ideally patients should receive the vaccine before their sexual debut. Nurses need to be able to address the fears, apprehensions, and misinformation among some parents and patients about the vaccine. Lastly, it is important for nurses to counsel all patients on the need for continued cervical cancer screening even for patients who have completed the vaccine series.

REFERENCES

1. Weinstock H, Berman S, Cates W Jr. Sexually transmitted diseases among American youth: incidence and prevalence estimates, 2000. Perspect Sex Reprod Health 2004;36(1):6–10.
2. Dempsey AF, Koutsky LA. National burden of genital warts: a first step in defining the problem. Sex Transm Dis 2008;35(4):361–2.
3. Dunne EF, Nielson CM, Stone KM, et al. Prevalence of HPV infection among men: a systematic review of the literature. J Infect Dis 2006;194(8):1044–57.
4. Dunne EF, Unger ER, Sternberg M, et al. Prevalence of HPV infection among females in the United States. JAMA 2007;297(8):813–9.
5. Weller Susan C, Stanberry, Lawrence R. Estimating the population prevalence of HPV. JAMA 2007;297(8):876–8.
6. Winer RL, Hughes JP, Feng Q, et al. Condom use and the risk of genital human papillomavirus infection in young women. N Engl J Med 2006;354(25):2645–54.
7. Bosch FX, de Sanjose S. Human papillomavirus and cervical cancer—burden and assessment of causality. J Natl Cancer Inst Monogr 2003;(31):3–13.
8. Winer RL, Lee S, Hughes JP, et al. Genital human papillomavirus infection: incidence and risk factors in a cohort of female university students. Am J Epidemiol 2003;157(3):218–26.
9. Moscicki A, Hills N, Shiboski S, et al. Risks for incident human papillomavirus infection and low-grade squamous intraepithelial lesion development in young females. JAMA 2001;285(23):2995–3002.
10. Ho GY, Bierman R, Beardsley L, et al. Natural history of cervicovaginal papillomavirus infection in young women. N Engl J Med 1998;338(7):423–8.
11. Roush S. MCIntyre L. Baldy L editors. Manual for the surveillance of vaccine-preventable diseases. Atlanta (GA): Centers for Disease Control and Prevention; 2008. No. 4.
12. National Institute of Health. Cervical cancer. NIH Consensus Statement 1996;14(1):1–38.
13. Palefsky JM, Holly EA. Immunosuppression and co-infection with HIV. J Natl Cancer Inst Monogr 2003;(31):41–6.
14. Castellsague X, Munoz N. Cofactors in human papillomavirus carcinogenesis—role of parity, oral contraceptives, and tobacco smoking. J Natl Cancer Inst Monogr 2003;(31):20–8.
15. Lowy DR, Frazer IH. Prophylactic human papillomavirus vaccines. J Natl Cancer Inst Monogr 2003;(31):111–6.

16. Joura EA, Leodolter S, Hernandez-Avila M, et al. Efficacy of a quadrivalent prophylactic human papillomavirus (types 6, 11, 16, and 18) L1 virus-like-particle vaccine against high-grade vulval and vaginal lesions: a combined analysis of three randomised clinical trials. Lancet 2007;369(9574):1693–702.
17. Joura EA, Kjaer SK, Wheeler CM, et al. HPV antibody levels and clinical efficacy following administration of a prophylactic quadrivalent HPV vaccine. Vaccine 2008;26(5):6844–51.
18. Center for Disease Control and Prevention. Human papillomavirus: HPV information for clinicans 2007. Available at: http://www.cdc.gov/std/HPV/STDFact-HPV-vaccine-hcp.htm.
19. Balog JE. The moral justification for a compulsory human papillomavirus vaccination program. Am J Public Health 2009;99(4):616–22.
20. Datta SD, Koutsky LA, Ratelle S, et al. Human papillomavirus infection and cervical cytology in women screened for cervical cancer in the United States, 2003-2005. Ann Intern Med 2008;148(7):493–500.
21. Singh G, Miller B, Hankkey B. Persistent area socioeconomic disparities in US incidence of cervical cancer, mortality, state and survival. Cancer 2004;101:1051–7.
22. Adams M, Jasani B, Fiander A. Human papilloma virus (HPV) prophylactic vaccination: challenges for public health and implications for screening. Vaccine 2007;25(16):3007–13.

The Role of Nursing in the Management of Unintended Pregnancy

Amy J. Levi, CNM, PhD, FACNM[a,*], Katherine E. Simmonds, RNC, MSN, MPH[b],
Diana Taylor, RN, PhD, FAAN[c]

KEYWORDS

- Unintended pregnancy • Reproductive health
- Reproductive health counseling
- Nursing's role in unintended pregnancy management
- Nursing advocacy in unintended pregnancy

The American Nurses Association Code of Ethics charges all nurses to "practice(s) with compassion and respect for the inherent dignity, worth and uniqueness of every individual, unrestricted by considerations of social or economic status, personal attributes, or the nature of health problems."[1] The identification of an unintended pregnancy may present a health problem that challenges the nurse's own belief systems and desire to support patient autonomy. It is imperative that nurses recognize that the health of women includes all aspects of their well-being, including attention to reproductive health concerns. Nurses have an ethical responsibility to consider women's needs for respectful and compassionate reproductive health care.

Nurses have been at the forefront of the protection and promotion of women's reproductive health since the beginning of the twentieth century, when Margaret Sanger, a nurse, took up the cause of a woman's right to control her fertility. A fearless, outspoken, and radical individual, Sanger's work led to the creation of the Planned Parenthood Federation of America, one of the largest women's health organizations in the United States. Margaret Sanger recognized that if women understood their reproductive cycles, they would be able to prevent pregnancy, and ultimately save themselves from the complications of self-induced abortions.[2] In this era of widely available contraception, it is hard to imagine a time when women did not have the ability to choose when they would conceive. It is equally difficult to appreciate that almost 100

[a] Department of Obstetrics/Gynecology and Reproductive Sciences, School of Medicine, University of California San Francisco, 1001 Potrero Avenue, 6D-29, San Francisco, CA 94110, USA
[b] Graduate Program in Nursing, Massachusetts General Hospital Institute of Health Professions, 36 1st Avenue, Charlestown, MA 02129, USA
[c] Department of Family Health Care Nursing, School of Nursing, University of California San Francisco, 2 Koret Way, N411Y, San Francisco, CA 94143, USA
* Corresponding author.
E-mail address: levia@obgyn.ucsf.edu (A. J. Levi).

Nurs Clin N Am 44 (2009) 301–314
doi:10.1016/j.cnur.2009.06.007   nursing.theclinics.com

years after the activism that produced both an array of contraceptive methods and their availability, women still become pregnant at a time they neither intend nor desire.

There are several reasons for nurses to focus on unintended pregnancy over other reproductive health issues. Unintended pregnancy is an extremely common occurrence in women's lives; at least half of all women in the United States will experience an unintended pregnancy by the age of 45 years.[3] Second, unintended pregnancy has negative consequences for the health of women and their children, and is associated with significant costs to the health care system.[4] On a positive note, meeting reproductive health needs, particularly for family planning services, is an important entry point into the heath care system for many women. Using these visits to address unintended pregnancy prevention can result in better health outcomes for women and their families. Finally, despite its frequency and significant costs, unintended pregnancy has received less attention—from research to the development of clinical care strategies—than other important health threats. This oversight can be attributed to the general fragmentation of health care services, as well as the politicization of reproductive health. These trends have contributed to the persistence of high rates of unintended pregnancy in the United States, which warrants the attention of all health professionals, including nurses.

NATIONAL HEALTH GOALS FOR REPRODUCTIVE HEALTH

Healthy People 2000 began as a public health compendium of national health goals, objectives, and tracking methods to be used as a road map for improving the health of all Americans. The nation's goal for unintended pregnancies as outlined in *Healthy People 2000* was a reduction in the rate of unintended pregnancies to 30% by the turn of the century. This goal was not met in 2000, and the rate of unintended pregnancy has remained stagnant at 50% over the past decade.[5]

Healthy People 2000 was redesigned in 2002 as *Healthy People 2010*, which includes 10 leading health indicators to assess the nation's health over the subsequent decade. Grounded in science, the *Healthy People 2010* national health indicators were selected because they motivate action, represent important public health issues, and can be measured to evaluate progress. The leading health indicators are physical activity, overweight/obesity, tobacco use, substance abuse, responsible sexual behavior, mental health, injury and violence, environmental quality, immunization, and access to health care. Improving responsible sexual behavior with the goal of improving pregnancy planning, preventing unintended pregnancy, and improving the health and well-being of women, infants, and families is the cornerstone of the national reproductive health goals in *Healthy People 2010*.[6] **Box 1** identifies the Family Planning Objectives included in *Healthy People 2010*.

PREVENTING AND MANAGING UNINTENDED PREGNANCY

Toward the goal of preventing and managing unintended pregnancy, the first *Healthy People 2000* objective proposed to increase the percentage of intended pregnancies to 70% by 2000.[7] However, nearly half of all pregnancies in the United States were unintended in 2002, giving the United States one of the highest unintended pregnancy rates in the industrialized world.[5] (A birth is classified as unintended if the mother says that, at the time of conception, she wanted to have the child later or wanted to have no more children. For the purposes of these statistics, all pregnancies ending in abortion were assumed to have been unintended.[8,9]) Of the approximately 6.4 million pregnancies in the United States in 2001, 3.1 million were unintended. Of these, approximately 1.4 million resulted in births, 1.3 million in abortions, and 430,000 in miscarriages. Although

---

Box 1
Healthy people 2010 objectives: family planning

9.1 Increase the proportion of pregnancies that are intended from 51% (1995) to 70%

9.2 Reduce the proportion of births occurring within 24 months of a previous birth from 11% (1995) to 6%

9.3 Increase the proportion of females at risk of unintended pregnancy (and their partners) who use contraception from 93% (1995) to 100%

9.4 Reduce the proportion of females experiencing pregnancy despite use of a reversible contraceptive method from 13% (1995) to 7%

9.5 Increase the proportion of health care providers who provide emergency contraception

9.6 Increase male involvement in pregnancy prevention and family planning efforts

9.7 Reduce pregnancies among adolescent females from 68 pregnancies/1000 females aged 15 to 17 years (1996) to 43 pregnancies/1000 females

9.8 Increase the proportion of adolescents who have never engaged in sexual intercourse before age 15 years from 81% (1995) to 88%

9.9 Increase the proportion of adolescents who have never engaged in sexual intercourse from 62% (1995) to 75%

9.10 Increase the proportion of sexually active, unmarried adolescents aged 15 to 17 years who use contraception that both effectively prevents pregnancy and provides barrier protection against disease

Data from US Department of Health and Human Services. Healthy people 2010: understanding and improving health. 2nd edition. Washington, DC: US Government Printing Office; 2000.

---

some unintended pregnancies are continued, almost half (48%) end in abortion. Approximately 1 in 20 women of reproductive age had an unintended pregnancy in 2001.[5,10]

There has been no substantial progress in meeting the target for this major reproductive health goal. Although unintended pregnancy rates have declined for middle- and upper-class women, rates are rising among the most socially disadvantaged women.[5,10] Unintended pregnancy rates in 2001 were substantially higher than among other groups for women aged 18 to 24, unmarried (particularly cohabiting) women, low-income women, women who did not complete high school, and minority women. In 2001, poor women had more than double the national average for unintended pregnancy (112 per 1000 women 15–44 years old), were five times as likely to have an unintended birth, and more than three times as likely to have an abortion as their higher-income counterparts.[10]

Consequences of the decision to continue an unintended pregnancy and to parent a child include several adverse effects. Unintended pregnancy is associated with a greater risk of birth defects, later entry into prenatal care, a lower number of total prenatal visits, tobacco and alcohol use during pregnancy, low birth weight, infant mortality, child abuse, and insufficient resources for child development.[8] Unintended pregnancy that results in a live birth is associated with physical abuse and violence during pregnancy and the 12 months before conception.[11]

In addition to measurable negative health consequences, the economic impact of unintended pregnancies is sizable: in 2002, the direct health care costs of unintended pregnancy were estimated to be 5 billion dollars. In contrast, the medical care savings associated with contraceptive use were estimated at 19 billion dollars for the same period.[4] Prevention of unintended pregnancy clearly is cost-effective, an important consideration during economically challenging times.

Screening, counseling, and preventive services have been found to be effective methods for meeting national health goals. The US Preventive Services Task Force (USPSTF), first convened by the Public Health Service in 1985, rigorously evaluates clinical research to assess the merits of preventive measures, including screening tests, counseling, immunizations, and preventive medications.[12] These primary and secondary preventive service recommendations, originally intended to inform primary care clinicians, now provide definitive standards for preventive services as well as providing health care quality measures for meeting national health objectives.

In the second edition of the *Guide to Clinical Preventive Services*,[13] a portion of the evidence reviewed indicated that a combination of patient education and access to effective contraception could reduce unintended pregnancy. Periodic counseling about effective contraceptive methods was recommended for all women and men at risk for unintended pregnancy and given a "B" recommendation (A rating of "A" or "B" reflects the highest magnitude of net benefit as well as the highest level of evidence supporting the provision of specific preventive service whereas a rating of "I" indicates insufficient evidence and a "D" rating recommends against a specific preventive service).[13] In the 1996 Preventive Services Guide, specific clinical guidelines for all sexually active adults and adolescents were included and recommended. However, despite the continuing high rate of unintended pregnancy, especially among minority and low-income women, primary and secondary preventive service guidelines related to unintended pregnancy have not been evaluated or included in subsequent guides. In contrast, most of the preventive services guidelines receiving A or B recommendations that are linked to national health goals have been regularly updated.[12]

In recent years, advances in prevention and the technology of early detection and management of unintended pregnancies have demonstrated improved safety and efficacy. Not only are these improvements not reflected in prevention guidelines, other evidence-based clinical practice guidelines for the prevention and comprehensive management of unintended pregnancy are virtually nonexistent. A review of the Agency for Health care Research and Quality National Guideline Clearinghouse identifies existing clinical practice guidelines that are narrowly focused on only a few components of unintended pregnancy prevention and management. For example, in the National Guideline Clearinghouse, the only practice guidelines relevant to this health issue are "Sexuality Education and Contraceptive Choices for Adolescents and Young People" and "Medical Management of Abortion." In addition, outdated guidelines are referenced for Unintended Pregnancy Counseling for Adults and Adolescents including Emergency Contraception.[13] Preconception care is one of the few aspects of unintended pregnancy prevention for which current evidence-based care models exist.

New advances have made earlier and simpler prevention and management of pregnancy possible, and appropriate for integration into primary care practice. Yet these advances have not translated into comprehensive, coordinated clinical processes to guide health professionals in the prevention and management of early unintended pregnancy. The politicization of sexuality across society, which extends to unintended pregnancy prevention and care, has resulted in fragmentation of services and a decline in access to coordinated care within primary care networks.

STRATEGIES TO PREVENT AND MANAGE UNINTENDED PREGNANCY: THE ROLE OF NURSING

In addition to a fragmented system for preventing and managing unintended pregnancies, there is also an overall lack of comprehensive sexuality education in the United States. As a result, many women do not fully understand how the reproductive system works, causing an underestimation of their true risk of pregnancy whether planned or unplanned. This lack of knowledge combines with a cultural unease among health professionals about discussing sexual topics, limited time for health care appointments, and the lack of a coordinated system of clinical guidelines and strategies for unintended pregnancy prevention that results in a system-wide failure to successfully provide care to women at risk of unintended pregnancy. As providers of care across multiple settings and the largest single group of health care providers, nurses have enormous potential to contribute to the realization of these national health goals related to unintended pregnancy and reproductive health.

There are numerous strategies for policy and practice that can improve access to quality reproductive health services and contribute to the prevention of unintended pregnancy; here the focus is on several that specifically involve nurses. These strategies can be categorized according to: (1) normalizing contraceptive and abortion services into a prevention framework; (2) addressing the role of nursing education in advancing nursing care competencies in reproductive health; and (3) encouraging and supporting reproductive health advocacy within the nursing profession. Each of these categories is described in the discussion that follows.

NORMALIZING CONTRACEPTIVE AND ABORTION SERVICES INTO A PREVENTIVE FRAMEWORK IN WOMEN'S HEALTH CARE

Normalizing contraceptive and abortion services into a preventive framework that is integrated into the broader health system is one strategy in which nursing can play an important role. Clinical practice guidelines, when developed by professional consensus and based on systematically reviewed and developed evidence, can provide a model for quality care. However, no comprehensive evidence-based clinical practice guidelines currently exist for the prevention and management of unintended pregnancy. Such guidelines ideally would address screening and management of early unintended pregnancy using organized, systematic primary, secondary, and tertiary prevention strategies.

Public health solutions to national health problems require primary, secondary, and tertiary prevention strategies. Primary prevention consists of health care services, medical tests, counseling, and health education and other actions designed to prevent the onset of targeted condition. Routine immunization of healthy individuals is a general example of primary prevention.[6] Primary prevention for unintended pregnancy should focus on activities before pregnancy to increase the chance that a pregnancy is desired and planned. These primary prevention strategies include preconception counseling; contraception counseling, dispensing and prescribing; and emergency contraception prescribing and dispensing.

Secondary prevention strategies are measures such as health care services designed to identify or treat individuals who have a disease or risk factors for a disease but who are not yet experiencing symptoms of the disease. Pap tests and high blood pressure screening are general examples of secondary prevention. Secondary prevention strategies for unintended pregnancy prevention are implemented once a pregnancy is detected. Essential prevention activities at this level include the following: pregnancy diagnostics (pregnancy tests, ultrasound) including screening for ectopic pregnancy and early pregnancy loss; pregnancy options counseling to support a woman to choose to continue a pregnancy, adoption, or abortion; referral and support for any decision reached following counseling to continue an unintended pregnancy and parent, adopt, or choose pregnancy termination; and pregnancy termination counseling for medication or aspiration abortion. For advanced practice nurses, this may include performance of medication or aspiration abortion depending on state regulations and professional practice guidelines, and postabortion care and follow-up, which may include psychosocial support or counseling and contraception counseling.

Tertiary prevention is represented by preventive health care measures or services that are part of the treatment and management of persons with clinical illnesses. Examples of tertiary prevention include cholesterol reduction in patients with coronary heart disease and insulin therapy to prevent complications of diabetes. Tertiary prevention in women with unintended pregnancy includes late term pregnancies requiring psychosocial care and support to women and their families continuing the pregnancy, adoption counseling, referral, and support, and second trimester abortion for women requiring termination.

Preconception Counseling

Because a woman's intentions concerning pregnancy affect both maternal risk behaviors and infant outcomes, planning a potential pregnancy is an essential component of primary prevention and women's reproductive health.[14] To achieve the *Healthy People 2010* objectives for reducing unintended pregnancy as well as other maternal and child health goals, a focus on preconception as well as perinatal health promotion has been recognized as an appropriate part of women's health care by the American Academy of Pediatrics,[15] the American College of Obstetricians and Gynecologists (ACOG),[16] the Association of Women's Health, Obstetric, and Neonatal Nurses (AWHONN),[17] the March of Dimes,[14] and others.

Preconceptual refers not only to women who are planning their first baby but can actually be applied to any period of time when a potentially fertile woman is not pregnant. Preconception care has evolved from being a specific entity to a health-promotion expectation of every professional providing care to any woman of childbearing capability. Preconception health promotion uses a prevention framework for every interaction with all women of childbearing potential. Nurses have made significant contributions to the development and provision of preconception health promotion and risk reduction activities.[15,18,19] All nurses who work with women of reproductive age (whether directly, through women's health care, or indirectly, in education and outreach to mothers of infants) must become competent in preconception health promotion. Special visits are not necessary to provide preconception health promotion.[14] For most women, counseling based on their personal profiles can be integrated into routine visits. This integration is likely to result in higher levels of personal wellness as well as an increase in intended, healthy pregnancies and healthy infants.

Every routine primary or specialty care visit and family planning visit (especially those that include a negative pregnancy test) is an opportunity to provide preconception care for health promotion, disease prevention, and reduction of prenatal and neonatal complications.[20] A major goal of preconception primary prevention is to provide counseling to delay pregnancy until the risks for poor pregnancy outcomes can be reduced. Preconceptual counseling can help a woman improve her lifestyle and health habits, and consider the responsibilities of carrying a pregnancy. Counseling about effective contraceptive use includes how an optimal pregnancy outcome is correlated with its intent and the woman's ability to prepare in advance. Other evidence-based practices for preconception counseling include the assessment of personal health risk factors, screening tests, and preventive health services, including all of the following:

- Review menstrual cycle physiology and educate about menstrual and ovulatory recording
- Review contraceptive use and contingency planning

- Review toxic exposures such as tobacco, alcohol, illicit or prescription medications, and potentially toxic chemicals or radiation
- Review nutritional and physical activity, immunization status, and psychosocial status
- Review medical and family history of patient and partner including sexually transmitted or other infections, genetic abnormalities, and serious conditions such as diabetes
- Screen for human immunodeficiency virus (HIV), hepatitis B, bacterial vaginosis, and other sexually transmissible infections
- Screen for genetic diseases and diabetes
- Supplement with at least 400 μg of folic acid daily to avoid birth defects
- Counsel about domestic violence, smoking cessation, and alcohol misuse
- Counsel about avoiding elevated body temperature (hot tubs) or fever from viruses and uncommon infectious organisms (eg, toxoplasmosis, salmonella)[21]

Opportunities for preconception health promotion can be integrated into all clinical settings in which nurses provide care. Some situations provide "teachable moments," when education and counseling about optimal pregnancy and pregnancy prevention is likely to be relevant to the patient.[22] These moments can occur following a negative pregnancy test result, diagnosis and treatment of a reproductive tract abnormality or infection, identification of a possible risk of infection with HIV or other sexually transmitted infections, identification of a substance abuse problem, or diagnosis of a significant medical problem.

Negative pregnancy test visits are a common and underexploited opportunity for primary prevention of unintended pregnancy. As many as one-quarter of all adolescent girls who conceive have had one or more visits to learn that their pregnancy test was negative.[23] Nurses who provide care to women and men of reproductive age in other clinical settings can also incorporate preconception health screening and health promotion strategies into their practice. In providing care to patients with chronic diseases such as hypertension, diabetes, depression, heart disease, autoimmune disease, epilepsy, asthma, or renal disease, both unintended pregnancy prevention and preconception health promotion can be addressed. Essential prevention strategies also include screening for hypertension, diabetes, and medications that are detrimental to fetal growth. Male partners' risk factors and the opportunity for pregnancy and infection prevention with male patients should also not be overlooked.

Nurses have been at the forefront in the development of resources for preconception health promotion, preconception risk assessment, and primary prevention strategies. In the Clinical Issues section of the *Journal of Obstetric, Gynecologic and Neonatal Nursing*, the scientific journal of the Association of Women's Health, Obstetric, Gynecologic and Neonatal Nursing, Merry K Moos[24] and other nursing leaders in reproductive health provide the evidence base for preconception health care.[15,20,25,26] Other resources in primary prevention of unintended pregnancy[27,28] and preconception health promotion for women's health care providers include evidence-based publications from AWHONN,[15] the March of Dimes,[14] and ACOG.[16] A central component of preconception health promotion is unintended pregnancy prevention through contraceptive counseling and management. An overview of this primary prevention strategy for nurses follows in the next section.

Contraception Counseling and Management

Efforts to decrease the likelihood of unintended pregnancies have focused on fertility prevention and improving contraceptive use. Research shows that almost half of women (48%) with an unintended pregnancy in 2001 used a contraceptive method during the month they became pregnant, as did 54% of those who had abortions.[5] Those who do use contraception still face some risk of unintended pregnancy because all methods have a statistical failure rate, or their use of their chosen method is imperfect.

All nurses should be competent in the basics of contraceptive management, which includes counseling related to fertility prevention goals, instruction on contraceptive regimen initiation and adherence, provision of a backup method, and information about emergency contraception. In addition, all nurses should use evidence-based, culturally competent, and lifespan-appropriate guidelines for counseling women and their families. Advanced practice nurses who care for women and their partners who are at risk for unintended pregnancy may also prescribe contraceptive methods, manage problems, and provide supportive counseling to help women negotiate contraceptive issues within their relationships. An overview of the evidence for including contraceptive counseling as part of all health encounters for women and men at risk for unintended pregnancy is provided later in this article. Full discussion of contraceptive counseling and management guidelines can be found in selected publications and online resources.

Contraception counseling has been shown to be effective to decrease inconsistency and misuse of available contraceptive methods. In a 2001 study of 900 women aged 18 to 44 years, personalized counseling as opposed to no counseling or only informational counseling significantly increased the odds of satisfaction with counseling, current contraceptive use, and intent to use contraception in the following year if at risk for an unintended pregnancy.[29] However, a 2003 review of studies published in English between 1985 and early 2000 found almost no experimental or observational literature that could reliably answer whether counseling in the clinical setting could impact unintended pregnancies.[28] A subsequent Cochrane Systematic Review examining randomized clinical trials and determined that, whereas good personal communication between clients and providers is generally considered important for successful use of hormonal contraception, little high-quality research exists that demonstrates enhanced counseling improves contraceptive use.[30] However limited the existing research, some small, well-conducted studies serve to guide patient interactions to improve contraceptive use. In addition, these findings suggest that contraceptive counseling should be included in all encounters with women and men at risk for unintended pregnancy.

In general, patient-centered counseling (ie, encouraging patients to ask questions, to participate in decision making, and to take part in self-care) has been found to improve health outcomes.[31] The USPSTF provides guidelines for clinicians regarding effective counseling interventions, and recommends that health care providers use every patient interaction as an opportunity to provide prevention-related and health counseling and education.[12] Moos[14] has proposed counseling methods for involving patients in contraceptive decision making as well as guidelines for health professionals to help women achieve their contraceptive goals. Moos[14] outlines four questions to engage a woman in considering a plan for preventing an unintended or mistimed pregnancy:

1. How many (more) children, if any, do you hope to have?
2. How long would you like to wait until you become pregnant (again)?
3. What do you plan to do to delay becoming pregnant until then?
4. What can I do to help you achieve your plan?

Counseling approaches for contraceptive users should include assessment, information, and strategies for successful contraceptive adherence.[14] Approaches that have been found to mobilize a patient's own decision and implement her intentions include the following:

- Assessment of the patient's understanding of the method and specific concerns. Ask questions such as: What experiences has she or her friends and family members previously had with the method? What has she heard about advantages or problems with the method?
- Inform the patient about potential side effects, their transient nature, and options available should the patient experience a problem. Dispel method misinformation and discuss noncontraceptive benefits.
- Contingency planning should be an important part of counseling. Clear, simple, and written guidance on what to do if the best intentions are not realized should be included with every contraceptive prescription. Every woman who is likely to have intercourse and who does not desire to become pregnant should be given anticipatory instructions on how to access and use emergency contraception (along with a prescription, if appropriate).[22]
- Link contraceptive counseling with counseling for prevention of sexually transmitted infections (STIs) for all sexually active adolescents and adults who have multiple current sexual partners. The USPSTF[32] now recommends high-intensity behavioral counseling to prevent STIs for all sexually active adolescents and for adults at increased risk for STIs.

Pregnancy Diagnostics and Options Counseling

All nurses should be able to appropriately evaluate individuals who present requesting a pregnancy test, or who are identified as at risk of pregnancy during a clinical encounter, and be able to provide counseling that is relevant to the results of that assessment.[33] In discussing options counseling, pregnancies that have been identified late in the pregnancy may present special needs for patients, including support and care for pregnancies that are going to be continued, adoption counseling and referrals, or care for women who decide to terminate.

THE ROLE OF NURSING EDUCATION IN ADVANCING NURSING CARE COMPETENCIES IN REPRODUCTIVE HEALTH

Despite the frequency of unintended pregnancy and abortion, many nursing, nurse practitioner, and nurse-midwifery programs do not adequately prepare students to care for these women, or teach about the most effective means of secondary prevention. Factors such as lack of faculty qualified to teach about reproductive options, fear of antichoice backlash, and the absence of appropriate didactic materials have been identified as barriers to incorporating this important subject into existing curricula.[34]

Another strategy for addressing the national health goals regarding unintended pregnancy is to make education about the prevention of unintended pregnancy a standard component of professional and nursing education in all accredited institutions. All women's health care professionals should learn to provide pregnancy options and abortion counseling. Training in abortion care should also be readily available to all.

Nursing students need to be made aware that in the ethical framework of the nursing profession, the decision to continue or terminate a pregnancy belongs to the pregnant woman. An individual provider's religious or moral beliefs must not impair the quality of health care available to a patient. Statutory "conscience clauses" and "refusal clauses" pertaining to health care providers must not be allowed to deny or impair the access of women or men to legal reproductive health services, procedures, and medications.[35]

Health care providers who do not provide contraceptive counseling or methods, pregnancy options counseling, or abortion referrals or services because of their personal moral or religious stance have a professional obligation to provide their patients with a timely referral to another health professional known to provide such services.

Some specific actions for advancing nursing education in the area of reproductive health include expanding innovative programs such as the Reproductive Options Education (ROE) Consortium for Nursing.[36] The ROE Consortium fills a critical void in nursing education by providing training, materials, support, and leadership to promote reproductive options in the curricula of nursing programs nationwide. By improving the training of nursing students, this project ultimately will advance quality and access to comprehensive reproductive health services for women and girls across the country.

Another specific action is to develop partnerships between nursing programs and reproductive health-focused professional or advocacy organizations to support and promote the integration of content on unintended pregnancy prevention and management, and facilitate training opportunities. Examples of existing partnerships include Clinicians for Choice and the Abortion Access Project, both of which are actively engaged with nurses, nurse educators, and nursing organizations and educational programs.[37] The Association of Reproductive Health Professionals (ARHP), an interdisciplinary organization representing health professionals and reproductive health advocates, has also developed an extensive Reproductive Health Education Curriculum that features peer-reviewed, evidence-based tools for health professions educators to use in their efforts to teach students about unintended pregnancy prevention and management, as well as other related reproductive health issues.[38] Further development of these existing partnerships, as well as the creation of new ones, will be essential for nursing to successfully integrate unintended pregnancy care into the core competencies of the profession.

Nursing faculty can also be influential in promoting reproductive rights and health in curriculum and educational policy. For example, the faculty of the Nurse-Midwifery and Women's Health Nurse Practitioner Program at the University of Illinois at Chicago support the international definition of reproductive health that "all people have the right to decide freely and responsibly the number and spacing of their children, and to have the information, education and means to do so; and the right to make decisions concerning reproduction free of discrimination, coercion and violence."[39] This definition provides the foundation for educational requirements for students in the program, as their policy on this subject states: "[w]hile individuals may have beliefs that differ, students are required to learn the full range of reproductive options available to women throughout the world and be able to counsel and refer women appropriately."[40] Other nursing programs could adopt similar educational policies that would further support the normalization of unintended pregnancy prevention and abortion as essential aspects of the care of women of reproductive age.

Nursing educators have been at the forefront in developing reproductive health curriculum and core competencies for women's health practice. Their dedication to high-quality education can continue by aligning educational curriculum and core competencies in women's and reproductive health with those for unintended pregnancy prevention including abortion care. To this end additional action steps that nurse educators can take include:

1. Situate abortion care curriculum within a broader public health model of unintended pregnancy prevention and management. At present, most programs teach primary prevention of unintended pregnancy such as preconception counseling, family

planning, and contraception skills including emergency contraception. As described in the previous section, secondary prevention of unintended pregnancy is focused on knowledge and skills of pregnancy diagnosis, pregnancy options counseling, and early abortion care, and tertiary care is focused on the care of women who present with unintended pregnancies at later gestational ages. It is these secondary and tertiary prevention components of unintended pregnancy that need development and incorporation into nursing education and training.

2. Specify core competencies for unintended pregnancy prevention and management across primary, secondary, and tertiary prevention competencies. For Advanced Practice Nursing faculty, this can mean the specification of Women's Health Core Competencies.[41]

3. Integrate core competencies into curriculum. Establish clinical opportunities for learning medication or aspiration abortion for basic and advanced practice nursing students.

REPRODUCTIVE HEALTH ADVOCACY WITHIN THE NURSING PROFESSION

There are many factors related to unintended pregnancy prevention beyond actual patient-provider encounter that nurses can influence. Some of these are barriers to contraceptive access due to insurance restrictions, conscience clauses making it possible for employers purchasing insurance packages to eliminate contraceptives as a covered service, and refusal of providers to prescribe, furnish, or dispense contraceptives including emergency contraception. In addition, regulation that limits or prohibits access to contraceptives services for minors, especially emergency contraception and abortion services, does not support reduction of unintended pregnancy, and may pose unnecessary health risks to young women and their families. As recently as 2007, the Centers for Disease Control reported that 48% of high school students had ever had sexual intercourse, and 15% of high school students had had four or more sex partners during their life, emphasizing the imperative for education and counseling for this high-risk population.[42]

Advocacy is an important activity for nurses, particularly in regard to the issue of access to reproductive services. The Nursing Code of Ethics and position statements from organizations such as the National Association of Nurse Practitioners in Women's Health (NPWH) and the ARHP can help to clarify the professional responsibilities of nurses. However, nurses need to work collectively to help clarify their ethical responsibilities through such efforts as the development of online continuing education programs, professional guidelines for advocacy, and tools for operationalizing ethical responsibilities related to reproductive rights.

Examples of advocacy activities address several actions, which include updating official statements from professional nursing organizations that focus on the public health issues related to unintended pregnancy discussed here. Professional nursing organizations can also work toward developing position papers or resolutions on the role of nursing education to support patient education on family planning and reproductive health. A third activity is to engage support organizations, such as Clinicians for Choice, in identifying nurses and primary care providers to become competent in reproductive options counseling, referral procedures, postabortion care, and the integration of unintended pregnancy prevention strategies into women's primary care.

The consequences of not addressing the public health costs of unintended pregnancy will only increase over time. Nurses have a fundamental role in preventing unwanted pregnancies and responding to them when they occur. In addition to clinical care, the nursing profession needs to address the prevention of unintended pregnancy through improvement in the quality of educational tools that address unintended pregnancy. Most importantly, advocacy activities by professional nursing organizations can reinforce the importance of the role of nursing education, clinical counseling, and regulatory support of nursing activities, which can ensure that families are able to have desired and healthy pregnancies.

REFERENCES

1. American Nurses Association. Code of ethics for nurses with interpretive statements. Available at: http://nursingworld.org/ethics/code/protected_nwcoe813. htm. Accessed March 2, 2009.
2. Gray M, Sanger M. A biography of the champion of birth control. New York: Richard Marek Publishers; 1979.
3. Jones RK, Singh S, Finer LB, et al. Repeat abortion in the United States. Occasional report. New York: Guttmacher Institute; 2006. No. 29.
4. Trussell J, Lalla AM, Doan QV, et al. Cost effectiveness of contraceptives in the United States. Contraception 2009;79(1):5–14.
5. Finer LB, Henshaw SK. Disparities in rates of unintended pregnancy in the United States, 1994 and 2001. Perspect Sex Reprod Health 2006;38(2):90–6.
6. Office of Population Affairs, Dept. Health and Human Services. Healthy people 2010—reproductive health. Available at: http://www.hhs.gov/opa/pubs/hp2010/ hp2010_rh.pdf. Accessed December 2008.
7. U.S. Department of Health and Human Services. Healthy people 2010: understanding and improving health. 2nd edition. Washington, DC: U.S. Government Printing Office; 2000.
8. Chandra A, Martinez GM, Mosher WD, et al. Fertility, family planning, and reproductive health of U. S. women: data from the 2002 National Survey on Family Growth. National Center for Vital Health Statistics. Vital Health Stat 2005;23(25).
9. Brown SS, Eisenberg L. From the Institute of Medicine. JAMA 1995;1274(17): 1332.
10. Santelli J, Rochat R, Hatfield-Timachy K, et al. The measurement and meaning of unintended pregnancy. Perspect Sex Reprod Health 2003;35(2):94–101.
11. Goodwin MM, Gazmararian JA, Johnson CH, et al. Pregnancy intendedness and physical abuse around the time of pregnancy: findings from the pregnancy risk assessment monitoring system, 1996–1997. Matern Child Health J 2000;4(2): 85–92.
12. US Preventive Services Task Force. Guide to clinical preventive service. 7th edition. Periodic updates; 2008. Available at: http://www.ahrq.gov/clinic/uspstfix.htm. Accessed February 20, 2009.
13. US Preventive Services Task Force. Unintended pregnancy counseling. Available at: http://www.ahrq.gov/clinic/2ndcps/unpregn.pdf. Accessed February 20, 2009.
14. Moos MK. Preconceptual health promotion: a focus for women's wellness. 2nd edition. White Plains (NY): March of Dimes; 2003.
15. American Academy of Pediatrics/American College of Obstetricians and Gynecologists. Guidelines for perinatal care. 4th edition. Elk Grove Village (IL): American College of Obstetricians and Gynecologists; 1997.
16. American College of Obstetricians and Gynecologists. Preconception care. No. 205. Washington, DC: ACOG Technical Bulletin; 1995.
17. Hobbins D. Full circle: the evolution of preconception health promotion in America. J Obstet Gynecol Neonatal Nurs 2003;32(4):516–22.

18. Cefalo RC, Moos MK. Preconceptual health care: a practical guide. 2nd edition. St. Louis (MO): Mosby; 1995.
19. Hobbins-Garbett D. Preconception counseling. In: Buttaro TM, Trybulski J, Bailey PP, editors. Primary care: a collaborative practice. St. Louis (MO): Mosby; 2000. p. 682–6.
20. Cullum AS. Changing provider practices to enhance preconceptual wellness. J Obstet Gynecol Neonatal Nurs 2003;32:543–9.
21. Hobbins D. Preconception care: maximizing the health of women and their newborns. Washington, DC: AWHONN; 2001.
22. Klein L, Stewart FH. Preconception care. In: Hatcher RA, Trussell J, Stewart F, et al, editors. Contraceptive technology. 18th edition. New York: Ardent Media; 2004. p. 617–28.
23. Zabin LS, Emerson MR, Ringers PA, et al. Adolescents with negative pregnancy test results. An accessible at-risk group. JAMA 1996;275(2):113–7.
24. Moos MK. Preconceptual wellness as a routine objective for women's health care: an integrative strategy. J Obstet Gynecol Neonatal Nurs 2003;32(4):550–6.
25. Postlethwaite D. Preconception health counseling for women exposed to teratogens: the role of the nurse. J Obstet Gynecol Neonatal Nurs 2003; 32(4):523–32.
26. Wallerstedt C, Lilley M, Baldwin K. Interconceptional counseling after perinatal and infant loss. J Obstet Gynecol Neonatal Nurs 2003;32(4):533–42.
27. Moos MK. Unintended pregnancies: a call for nursing action. MCN Am J Matern Child Nurs 2003;28(1):24–30.
28. Moos MK, Bartholomew N, Lohr K. Counseling in the clinical setting to prevent unintended pregnancy: an evidence-based research agenda. Contraception 2003;67:115–33.
29. Weisman CS, Maccannon DS, Henderson JT, et al. Contraceptive counseling in managed care: preventing unintended pregnancy in adults. Womens Health Issues 2002;12(2):79–95.
30. Henshaw S. Unintended pregnancy in the United States. Fam Plann Perspect 1998;30:24–9, 46.
31. Lipkin M Jr. Physician-patient interaction in reproductive counseling. Obstet Gynecol 1998;88:31S–40S.
32. US Preventive Services Task Force. Behavioral counseling to prevent sexually transmitted infections: recommendation statement. Available at: http://www. ahrq.gov/clinic/uspstf08/sti/stirs.htm. Accessed February 20, 2009.
33. Simmonds K, Likis F. Providing options counseling for women with unintended pregnancies. J Obstet Gynecol Neonatal Nurs 2005;34(3):373–9.
34. Foster AM, Polis C, Allee MK, et al. Abortion education in nurse practitioner, physician assistant and certified nurse-midwifery programs: a national survey. Contraception 2006;73(4):408–14.
35. Association of Reproductive Health Professionals. Abortion position statement. Available at: http://www.arhp.org/About-Us/Position-Statements#1. Accessed March 30, 2009.
36. The reproductive options education consortium for nursing. Available at: http:// www.abortionaccess.org/content/view/27/76/. Accessed March 30, 2009.
37. Clinicians for Choice. Available at: http://www.prochoice.org/cfc/. Accessed March 30, 2009.
38. Association for Reproductive Health Professionals. Available at: http://www.arhp. org/. Accessed March 30, 2009.

39. United Nations Department of Public Information. Summary of the ICPD Programme of Action. Available at: http://www.unfpa.org/icpd/summary.cfm#chapter2. Accessed March 30, 2009.

40. University of Illinois-Chicago Nurse Midwifery and Women's Health Nurse Practitioner Program. Ethical requirements for CNM/WHNP students. Chicago, 2003.

41. United States Department of Health and Human Services. Health Resources Service Administration, Bureau of Health Professions, Division of Nursing. Nurse practitioner primary care competencies in specialty areas: adult, family, gerontological, pediatric, and women's health. Available at: http://www.nonpf.com/finalaug2002.pdf. Accessed March 30, 2009.

42. CDC. Youth risk behavior surveillance—United States, 2007. MMWR Morb Mortal Wkly Rep 2008;57(SS-4):1–131.

Cardiac Health: Primary Prevention of Heart Disease in Women

Melanie Warziski Turk, PhD, MSN, RN[a],*, Patricia K. Tuite, MSN, RN[b],
Lora E. Burke, PhD, MPH, FAHA, FAAN[c]

KEYWORDS

- Heart disease • Prevention • Women • Lifestyle
- Evidence-based • Risk factors

Today, over 41 million women suffer from cardiovascular disease (eg, coronary heart disease, stroke, and congestive heart failure) in the United States, with more than 450,000 women dying each year. Coronary heart disease (CHD) is the leading cause of death in women 65 years of age and older. One out of every 6 female deaths is associated with CHD.[1] These are startling statistics, but more recently death rates among men have decreased by 52% and, among women 65 years and older, death rates have decreased by 49%.[2] Current research has helped explain the underlying contributions to these reductions in mortality. Evidence-based medical therapies have decreased death rates by 47%, and behavioral changes to alter risk factors have reduced death rates by 44%.[3] Therefore, a woman can decrease her CHD risk by targeting lifestyle habits.

The Nurses' Health Study is a large cohort study designed to assess the effects of a combination of lifestyle practices on the risk of coronary heart disease.[4–7] Findings from this longitudinal, observational study demonstrated that a woman was able to decrease the incidence of a coronary event by more than 80% through not smoking, maintaining normal body weight (body mass index [BMI; weight in kilograms divided by height in meters squared] <25 kg/m^2), consuming a healthy diet, participating in moderate to vigorous exercise for 30 minutes a day, and consuming a moderate amount of alcohol.[5,7] Over the 14-year period studied, the incidence of CHD declined

L.E.B.'s effort was partially supported by 1K24 NR010742.
[a] School of Nursing, Duquesne University, Fisher Hall 5th Floor, 600 Forbes Avenue, Pittsburgh, PA 15282, USA
[b] Department of Acute and Tertiary Care, School of Nursing, University of Pittsburgh, 360 Victoria Building, 3500 Victoria Street, Pittsburgh, PA 15261, USA
[c] Department of Health and Community Systems, School of Nursing, Graduate School of Public Health, University of Pittsburgh, 415 Victoria Building, 3500 Victoria Street, Pittsburgh, PA 15261, USA
* Corresponding author.
E-mail address: turkm@duq.edu (M.W. Turk).

by 31% across all age groups. Research has demonstrated that primary prevention can help decrease the incidence of CHD as well as the associated mortality rates. The purpose of this article is to describe the assessment of risk factors associated with CHD, present the current evidence on prevention of CHD, and discuss guidelines for implementing findings in practice.

ASSESSMENT OF RISK FACTORS
History

An important first step in assessing a woman's risk for CHD is to collect information on her medical, social, lifestyle, and family history. A thorough evaluation of the medical history including preexisting medical conditions, such as hypertension, dyslipidemia, and diabetes, is necessary to determine the woman's baseline risk. Patients with diabetes are at a higher risk for CHD and have 2 times the risk of myocardial infarction (MI) compared with the general population.[8] Elevated blood pressure and abnormal lipids are strong, independent risk factors for CHD.[9] Assessment of the social and lifestyle history provides information regarding behaviors, such as smoking, alcohol consumption, dietary habits, and physical activity. Smoking, obesity, a diet high in fat, and a sedentary lifestyle are all risk factors for heart disease.[10,11] Smoking is associated with a greater risk of MI in women, particularly among women less than 45 years of age.[12] Overweight and obesity are associated with comorbid conditions such as heart failure and increase one's risk for CHD and sudden death.[13] A longitudinal evaluation of more than 111,000 patients found that severely obese individuals (BMI ≥ 40 kg/m^2), which comprised about 6% of the sample, experienced their first MI 12 years sooner than their normal weight counterparts.[14] A sedentary lifestyle is associated with an increase in CHD risk and cardiovascular disease (CVD) mortality.[15] Patient information concerning these lifestyle habits is part of the overall assessment of baseline risk. Family history is another critical component that must be considered in determining risk for CVD. A woman who has a first-degree relative with premature CVD (ie, <55 years old in a male relative and <65 years old in a female relative) is considered at risk.[16]

Symptoms

Precordial or retrosternal chest pain or pressure is one of the classic symptoms of an MI. The quality of the pain has been described as heaviness, crushing, aching, burning, or squeezing, and has been noted to radiate to the jaw, neck, arms, or back. Other associated symptoms include shortness of breath, nausea/vomiting, diaphoresis, and lightheadedness. Research shows that about 33% of patients present without chest pain, and symptoms in women tend to be more atypical; for example, the absence of chest pain is more common in women than men.[17] Women also tend to present with more associated symptoms such as middle or upper back pain, neck or jaw pain, shortness of breath, indigestion, and fatigue.[17,18]

Physical Examination

A physical examination for the evaluation of risk should include blood pressure, BMI, and waist circumference (WC) as well as blood work (ie, fasting glucose and lipid profile). A normal systolic blood pressure is less than 120 mm Hg and a normal diastolic blood pressure is less than 80 mm Hg. A BMI between 18.5 and 24.9 kg/m^2 is normal weight, 25 to 29.9 kg/m^2 is overweight, and more than 30 kg/m^2 is considered obese.[13] The goal for the patient is to achieve a normal, healthy body weight. Increased WC, a measure of abdominal adiposity, has been correlated with increased risk of insulin resistance, diabetes, MI, and even death.[19,20] Sex-specific cutoffs have been established to identify relative risk; women with a WC more than 35 inches (88 cm) are at high risk for developing morbidities like CVD.[9] To measure WC, palpate the upper hipbone to locate the iliac crest, and draw a horizontal line just above the upper border of the iliac crest. Cross that line with a vertical line from the mid-axillary position. Keeping the measuring tape parallel to the floor, wrap the tape around the abdomen at the level of the marked point, and take the measurement during the patient's exhalation.[21] A blood glucose level should be measured after an 8-hour fast. A normal level is 100 mg/dL or less; a person is considered prediabetic with a blood glucose level of 101 to 125 mg/dL, and diabetes is present if the fasting level is 126 mg/dL or more.[22] Desirable fasting lipid profiles for women, drawn after a 12-hour fast, include low-density lipoprotein cholesterol (LDL-C) level less than 100 mg/dL, high-density lipoprotein cholesterol (HDL-C) level greater than 50 mg/dL, triglycerides level less than 150 mg/dL, and non-HDL-C (the total cholesterol minus HDL-C) level less than 130 mg/dL.[16]

Framingham Risk Assessment

Risk factor assessment provides the chance to identify asymptomatic women who are in danger of developing CHD in the long term. The Framingham Risk Score (FRS) is a tool that may be used to assess one's 10-year likelihood of MI or CHD death by assigning a point value to each of 5 established risk factors—age, total cholesterol, HDL-C, blood pressure, and cigarette smoking.[23] The total score is used to determine low risk (<10% risk of MI or CHD death), intermediate risk (10%–20% risk), or high risk (>20% risk).[9] Because overall lifetime risk for CVD approaches one in every two women[24] and this score is focused on 10-year risk, the FRS should be used as part of the total risk assessment that includes medical, lifestyle, and family history.[16]

EVIDENCE FOR PREVENTION
Dietary Intake

In the prevention of CHD, it is important to consume an overall healthy diet focusing on adequate nutrient intake and energy balance. Evidence-based recommendations from the American Heart Association (AHA) include balancing caloric intake with energy expenditure to attain or maintain a normal body weight (BMI <25 kg/m^2), eating a diet containing an abundance of fruits, vegetables, whole-grain and high-fiber foods, fish twice weekly, and moderate alcohol consumption.[11] In particular, fruits and vegetables that are rich in color (eg, dark green and orange) should be consumed several times a week. Whole grains include items like whole wheat, oats, corn, and brown rice, and should comprise a minimum of half an individual's grain intake. Fiber intake should be between 20 and 30 g/d.[9] Fish is recommended, particularly oily fish, because it is rich in long-chain w-3 polyunsaturated fatty acids, and is associated with a decreased risk of sudden death and death from CHD.[11] Moderate alcohol intake has been associated with a beneficial effect on cardiovascular health[25] and therefore, if individuals consume alcohol, no more than one drink per day is recommended for a woman. A large, international case control study found daily consumption of fruits and vegetables, moderate- or vigorous-intensity physical activity, and at least thrice weekly alcohol consumption to be protective against acute MI.[26]

Food items that should be restricted in a woman's diet include saturated fat, *trans* fat, cholesterol, added sugars, and salt.[11] The intake of saturated fat, *trans* fat, and cholesterol should be limited to less than 7% of fat intake, less than 1% of fat intake, and less than 300 mg, respectively. *Trans* fats are partially hydrogenated fats created by adding hydrogen to liquid vegetable oils, making the oils solid for use in bakery items, prepackaged snacks, and deep-fried foods.[27] To achieve these fat intake goals, women should consume lean meats or meat alternatives and dairy products that are fat-free or low-fat. Total dietary fat intake should not exceed 35% of total daily caloric intake.[9] Among the participants in the Nurses' Health Study, improvement in diet, (such as a 31% decline in the intake of *trans* fats and a 90% increase in the intake of cereal fiber) explained a 16% decrease in CHD between the assessment points of 1980 to 1982 and 1990 to 1992, after adjusting for age and smoking.[5] Limiting the intake of foods and beverages with added sugars is advocated to support lower caloric intake, energy balance, and adequate nutrient intake. Selecting and cooking foods with little salt can support blood pressure control and a daily limit of 2.3 g/d of sodium is recommended.[11] Because eating outside of the home is associated with larger food portions and food items of higher energy density and salt content, women should choose foods carefully when eating in restaurants and practice portion control.

Physical Activity

There has been significant research to support the use of exercise in decreasing the risk of CHD.[28–31] By improving overall fitness and increasing exercise capacity, one can decrease risk that may result in up to a 35% reduction in CHD.[28] Current recommendations to improve health, from the American College of Sports Medicine (ACSM) and the AHA, advise individuals between the ages of 18 and 65 years to participate in moderate-intensity aerobic physical activity for a minimum of 150 minutes per week or vigorous-intensity aerobic activity for at least 75 minutes per week.[32] A combination of moderate- and vigorous-intensity activity will yield the same benefits. Updated recommendations also suggest that individuals will benefit from twice-weekly activities that increase muscle strength (8–10 weight resistance exercises with 8–12 repetitions per exercise).

The Women's Health Initiative Observational Study enrolled 73,743 postmenopausal women to examine total physical activity score, walking, vigorous exercise, and hours spent sitting or sleeping as predictors of cardiovascular events.[29] The study found that the total physical activity score at baseline exhibited a strong inverse relationship with CHD. The more activity a woman participated in, the lower her risk for the development of disease. Women who exercised for 2.5 hours per week, by walking or through vigorous exercise, decreased their risk for CHD by 30%. This finding is consistent with the guidelines established by the AHA and the ACSM. Risk was decreased further if the women participated in both vigorous activity and walking than either one alone. Cardiovascular risk decreased less in women who spent more time sitting or lying compared with those who moved around more.[29]

Lee and colleagues[30] examined the relationship between physical activity, specifically walking, and the risk of CHD among women. Data indicated that at least 1 hour of walking per week predicted a lower risk for CHD. This study indicated that even light to moderate activity is associated with lower CHD rates in women. Women who participated in 600 to 1499 kcal/wk of physical activity had a significant decrease in coronary risk factors. When women in the highest level of physical activity were compared with women in the lowest category, data showed a lower risk of CHD among the women who were most active.[30]

Bassuk and Manson[31] also discussed the cardioprotective mechanisms associated with exercise. These investigators stated that exercise reduces cardiovascular risk independently of weight regulation. Thirty minutes of moderate-intensity activity has been shown to lower blood pressure, raise glucose tolerance and insulin sensitivity, and improve lipid levels. In summary, all of the findings indicated that walking and vigorous exercise were associated with a decrease in CHD events. By increasing physical activity to at least 150 minutes per week, a woman can decrease her risk for CHD.

Weight Management

Body weight management is critically important for promoting cardiac health because obesity is linked to cardiac arrhythmias, congestive heart failure, ischemic heart disease, and sudden death;[10] obesity was added as an independent risk factor for CHD more than 10 years ago.[33] For normal-weight women, weight gain should be avoided by ensuring a balance between energy consumed and energy expended, to prevent the average weight gain of 0.5 to 1 kg accumulated annually by adults in the United States.[34] Efforts to avoid the positive energy imbalance resulting in weight gain, which includes small reductions in food intake or increases in physical activity, may need to be intensified over a woman's lifetime to adjust for physiologic, age-related changes.[35] For women who are overweight or obese, the recommended initial weight loss goal is 10% of baseline weight[21] because losing and maintaining a moderate 10% weight loss is associated with improvement in insulin resistance, hypertension, dyslipidemia, and inflammation.[10] A weight loss program should include a 500 calorie per day reduction in food intake and a 1000 calorie per week expenditure in physical activity to obtain a weight loss of 0.5 to 1.0 kg per week.[36]

Behavioral approaches to the treatment of obesity include several common components: goal setting for dietary intake and physical activity, self-monitoring, problem solving, stimulus control, cognitive restructuring, and relapse prevention.[36,37] Goal setting involves setting daily and weekly targets for calorie and fat intake as well as physical activity, for example, consuming 1200 to 1500 calories daily, 25% of calories from fat, and engaging in 150 minutes of physical activity each week.[38,39] Self-monitoring requires keeping a detailed record of food intake and activity to increase one's awareness of behaviors that support or hinder weight loss endeavors,[36] and has consistently been associated with success in losing weight and maintaining weight loss.[40,41] Problem-solving techniques help individuals recognize barriers to their weight loss efforts, choose potential resolutions to these barriers, apply the solution, then examine the effectiveness. Using stimulus control, one modifies the environment to support behaviors that promote weight loss or maintenance, for example, placing fresh fruit or vegetables in visible places, placing high fat foods in the back of the cabinet, and placing athletic shoes by the door as a reminder to take a walk. Recognizing and adjusting weight control thoughts is accomplished through cognitive restructuring, like replacing negative or all-or-nothing thoughts with positive and self-affirming thoughts. In relapse prevention training, individuals are taught how to recognize high-risk situations for lapses in their behavior changes, for example, eating at parties and anticipating the challenges of staying with their eating plan. Individuals must also develop a plan for how they will manage high-risk situations, perhaps even role-playing the situation with the person counseling them.[36]

Pharmacotherapy is an appropriate weight loss tool for certain women and is currently approved for persons with a BMI of 30 kg/m^2 or more or for those with a BMI of 27 kg/m^2 or more who have obesity-related comorbidities (eg, sleep apnea, diabetes, hypertension). Two medications, sibutramine and orlistat, have been approved by the US Food and Drug Administration for up to 2 years of long-term use, and have been found to be beneficial for weight loss maintenance.[42] Sibutramine reduces appetite by blocking the reuptake of serotonin and noradrenaline in the central nervous system; 10 mg/d is the recommended initial dose. Sibutramine should be used cautiously in women with hypertension, stroke, and CVD due to the potential for increased heart rate and blood pressure.[10] Orlistat decreases fat absorption by approximately 30% at the 120 mg thrice daily dosage through gastrointestinal tract inhibition of gastric and pancreatic lipases essential for digestion of fats, but has been associated with side effects like oily stools or fecal incontinence, and decreased absorption of fat-soluble vitamins A, D, and E. A half-strength dosage of orlistat is available without a prescription as Alli. Drug therapy must be used in conjunction with lifestyle changes to be effective over the long term.[10]

Surgical treatment of obesity may be indicated in women with severe obesity (BMI $\geq$40 kg/m^2) or a BMI of 35 kg/m^2 or more and comorbidities like sleep apnea, diabetes, or hypertension.[43] Several bariatric surgical approaches are used for weight loss using restrictive or malabsorptive methods, for example, gastric bypass, vertical banded gastroplasty, adjustable gastric banding, and biliopancreatic diversion.[44] A meta-analysis of 22,094 patients that examined the impact of bariatric surgery found that diabetes and hypertension were resolved in 76.8% and 61.7% of patients, respectively; in at least 70% of patients, dyslipidemia improved.[45] After 10 years of follow-up, The Swedish Obese Subjects Study reported better recovery rates from diabetes, elevated triglycerides, hypertension, and low levels of HDL-C compared with matched control participants.[46] For the severely obese patient, weight loss induced by bariatric surgery is associated with an improvement in cardiovascular risk profile.

Smoking Cessation

Although there is limited evidence from randomized trials, it is still strongly recommended that women refrain from smoking or exposing themselves to second-hand smoke. Smoking cessation has been identified as an important lifestyle intervention in the prevention of CHD.[16,47] The Nurses' Health Study clearly demonstrated a decrease in coronary events through changes in lifestyle including smoking cessation. The risk of CHD declined by 31% across all age groups, and these results were consistent with a decrease in smoking by 41%.[5] Another prospective cohort study completed in Copenhagen, Denmark also found that there was a decrease in risk for MI when an individual quit smoking. There was no change in risk for individuals who only decreased the amount of cigarettes smoked per day.[48] Women should be encouraged to quit smoking to prevent CHD. There are many avenues available to assist with smoking cessation, including counseling, nicotine replacement, and other pharmacotherapies. Many of these therapies in conjunction with a formalized smoking cessation program that provides group counseling can help a woman to quit smoking.

Management of Hypertension and Dyslipidemia

A blood pressure less than 120/80 mm Hg is optimal for the prevention of CHD and can be accomplished through weight control, increasing physical activity, using alcohol in moderation, restricting sodium intake, and increasing the intake of fruits, vegetables, and low-fat dairy products.[16,47] If blood pressure is 140/90 mm Hg or greater, pharmacotherapy is indicated. Thiazide diuretics are used for most patients unless contraindicated. If a woman is considered to be at high-risk then β-blockers or the addition of an angiotensin-converting enzyme inhibitor along with a thiazide agent is recommended.[16]

Drug therapy along with lifestyle interventions, such as increasing physical activity, should be used in women with CHD to keep the LDL-C level below 100 mg/dL.[16,47] Aerobic exercise will increase HDL-C levels, thus decreasing risk.[49,50] If increasing physical activity and reducing body weight still does not decrease cholesterol levels, statins are effective in lowering LDL levels. Research has shown that statins can decrease the 5-year incidence of major coronary events.[51] Based on the aforementioned evidence, it is important for health care professionals to encourage women to make changes to control blood pressure and manage lipid levels to decrease CHD risk. **Table 1** gives a summary of modifiable risk factors for CHD.

NURSING IMPLICATIONS: IMPLEMENTING GUIDELINES INTO PRACTICE

Nurses need to assess CHD risk in female patients and recommend lifestyle changes to all women as appropriate. Lifestyle recommendations include smoking cessation, following a dietary pattern that is consistent with heart health, incorporating physical activity on a routine basis, and maintaining or losing weight to attain a BMI between 18.5 and 24.9 kg/m². If the person is overweight or obese, a 7% to 10% weight loss can reduce risk for diabetes and CHD.[52,53] A woman's perceived barriers to following these guidelines need to be assessed. Barriers to healthy eating, for example, concerns over taste, insufficient time, the belief that healthy foods cost more, and barriers to physical activity (eg, lack of time, motivation, costly exercise facilities), have been reported.[54] Additional barriers that nurses can focus on include women's confusion regarding mixed messages about heart health in the media, the misperception that heart health is not so important for women, and the view that providers do not explain exactly how a woman can alter her risk for CHD.[55] To help women achieve a healthy weight, nurses can access a document published in 2000, the *Practical Guide to the Identification, Evaluation, and Treatment of Overweight and Obesity in Adults,* available at http://www.nhlbi.nih.gov/guidelines/obesity/prctgd_c.pdf. This guide provides detailed information on assessing and treating the overweight or obese patient as well as specific patient educational tools, for example, how to read food labels, lower-calorie food alternatives, and sample reduced-calorie menus for different cuisine preferences.[56] Nurses are in a key position to provide oversight of the implementation of the guidelines to prevent CHD in women as well as support for and reinforcement of successful lifestyle modification promoting heart health.

Table 1
Modifiable risk factors for CHD prevention

Risk Factor	Recommendation
Weight	Balance caloric intake and energy expenditure to maintain BMI <25 kg/m². If overweight or obese, strive to reduce weight by 7%–10%, or prevent further weight gain
Sedentary lifestyle	Participate in at least 150 min of moderate to vigorous physical activity per week and exercise to increase muscle strength twice per week
Cigarette smoking	Smoking cessation
Hypertension	Maintain blood pressure <120/80 mm Hg through diet and exercise or the use of pharmacotherapy
Hyperlipidemia	Maintain LDL <100 mg/dL, HDL >50 mg/dL, and triglyceride levels <150 mg/dL through diet and exercise. Pharmacologic agents can be used as necessary

Data from Mosca L, Banka CL, Benjamin EJ, et al. Evidence-based guidelines for cardiovascular disease prevention in women: 2007 update. Circulation 2007;115(11):1481–501.

SUMMARY

CHD is the leading cause of death among women, and the risk greatly increases as a woman reaches menopause. Engaging in healthier behaviors including maintaining a healthy weight, leading a nonsedentary lifestyle, and refraining from smoking significantly decreases a woman's risk of developing CHD. Health care professionals are instrumental in assisting a woman to identify her risk factors by obtaining an in-depth history, a complete physical assessment, and determining risk through the use of assessment tools such as the Framingham risk assessment. Nurses can also assess a woman for any perceived barriers that prevent her from participating in an active lifestyle and maintaining a healthy diet. Heart disease can be prevented, and nurses can be instrumental in helping a woman make lifestyle changes to decrease her risk.

REFERENCES

1. Lloyd-Jones D, Adams R, Carnethon M, et al. Heart disease and stroke statistics—2009 update: a report from the American Heart Association Statistics Committee and Stroke Statistics Subcommittee. Circulation 2009;119(3): e21–181.
2. Ford ES, Capewell S. Coronary heart disease mortality among young adults in the U.S. from 1980 through 2002: concealed leveling of mortality rates. J Am Coll Cardiol 2007;50(22):2128–32.
3. Ford ES, Ajani UA, Croft JB, et al. Explaining the decrease in U.S. deaths from coronary disease, 1980-2000. N Engl J Med 2007;356(23):2388–98.
4. Manson JE, Hu FB, Rich-Edwards JW, et al. A prospective study of walking as compared with vigorous exercise in the prevention of coronary heart disease in women. N Engl J Med 1999;341(9):650–8.
5. Hu FB, Stampfer MJ, Manson JE, et al. Trends in the incidence of coronary heart disease and changes in diet and lifestyle in women. N Engl J Med 2000;343(8): 530–7.
6. Hu FB, Stampfer MJ, Solomon C, et al. Physical activity and risk for cardiovascular events in diabetic women. Ann Intern Med 2001;134(2):96–105.
7. Stampfer MJ, Hu FB, Manson JE, et al. Primary prevention of coronary heart disease in women through diet and lifestyle. N Engl J Med 2000;343(1):16–22.
8. Buse JB, Ginsberg HN, Bakris GL, et al. Primary prevention of cardiovascular diseases in people with diabetes mellitus: a scientific statement from the American Heart Association and the American Diabetes Association. Circulation 2007;115(1):114–26.
9. Expert Panel on Detection Evaluation and Treatment of High Blood Cholesterol in Adults. Executive summary of the third report of The National Cholesterol Education Program (NCEP) expert panel on detection, evaluation, and treatment of high blood cholesterol in adults (Adult Treatment Panel III). JAMA 2001;285(19): 2486–97.
10. Klein S, Burke LE, Bray GA, et al. Clinical implications of obesity with specific focus on cardiovascular disease. A statement for professionals from the American Heart Association Council on nutrition, physical activity, and metabolism. Circulation 2004;110:2952–67.
11. Lichtenstein AH, Appel LJ, Brands M, et al. Diet and lifestyle recommendations revision 2006: a scientific statement from the American Heart Association Nutrition Committee. Circulation 2006;114(1):82–96.

12. Njolstad I, Arnesen E, Lund-Larsen PG. Smoking, serum lipids, blood pressure, and sex differences in myocardial infarction. A 12-year follow-up of the Finnmark study. Circulation 1996;93(3):450–6.
13. Poirier P, Giles TD, Bray GA, et al. Obesity and cardiovascular disease: pathophysiology, evaluation, and effect of weight loss: an update of the 1997 American Heart Association scientific statement on obesity and heart disease from the obesity committee of the council on nutrition, physical activity, and metabolism. Circulation 2006;113(6):898–918.
14. Madala MC, Franklin BA, Chen AY, et al. Obesity and age of first non-ST-segment elevation myocardial infarction. J Am Coll Cardiol 2008;52(12):979–85.
15. Houde SC, Melillo KD. Cardiovascular health and physical activity in older adults: an integrative review of research methodology and results. J Adv Nurs 2002; 38(3):219–34.
16. Mosca L, Banka CL, Benjamin EJ, et al. Evidence-based guidelines for cardiovascular disease prevention in women: 2007 update. Circulation 2007;115(11): 1481–501.
17. Canto JG, Goldberg RJ, Hand MM, et al. Symptom presentation of women with acute coronary syndromes: myth vs reality. Arch Intern Med 2007;167(22): 2405–13.
18. McSweeney JC, Cody M, O'Sullivan P, et al. Women's early warning symptoms of acute myocardial infarction. Circulation 2003;108(21):2619–23.
19. Yusuf S, Hawken S, Ounpuu S, et al. Obesity and the risk of myocardial infarction in 27,000 participants from 52 countries: a case-control study. Lancet 2005; 366(9497):1640–9.
20. Pischon T, Boeing H, Hoffmann K, et al. General and abdominal adiposity and risk of death in Europe. N Engl J Med 2008;359(20):2105–20.
21. NHLBI obesity education initiative expert panel on the identification evaluation and treatment of overweight and obesity. Clinical guidelines on the identification, evaluation, and treatment of overweight and obesity in adults: the evidence report. Obes Res 1998;6(Suppl 2):S51–S209.
22. American Diabetes Association. Available at: http://www.diabetes.org/. Accessed March 27, 2009.
23. Wilson PWF, D'Agostino RB, Levy D, et al. Prediction of coronary heart disease using risk factor categories. Circulation 1998;97(18):1837–47.
24. Lloyd-Jones DM, Leip EP, Larson MG, et al. Prediction of lifetime risk for cardiovascular disease by risk factor burden at 50 years of age. Circulation 2006; 113(6):791–8.
25. Flesch M, Rosenkranz S, Erdmann E, et al. Alcohol and the risk of myocardial infarction. Basic Res Cardiol 2001;96(2):128–35.
26. Yusuf S, Hawken S, Ounpuu S, et al. Effect of potentially modifiable risk factors associated with myocardial infarction in 52 countries (the INTERHEART study): case-control study. Lancet 2004;364(9438):937–52.
27. Mozaffarian D, Katan MB, Ascherio A, et al. Trans fatty acids and cardiovascular disease. N Engl J Med 2006;354(15):1601–13.
28. Thompson PD, Buchner D, Pina IL, et al. Exercise and physical activity in the prevention and treatment of atherosclerotic cardiovascular disease: a statement from the Council on Clinical Cardiology (Subcommittee on Exercise, Rehabilitation, and Prevention) and the Council on Nutrition, Physical activity, and Metabolism (Subcommittee on Physical Activity). Circulation 2003;107(24): 3109–16.

29. Manson JE, Greenland P, LaCroix AZ, et al. Walking compared with vigorous exercise for the prevention of cardiovascular events in women. N Engl J Med 2002;347(10):716–25.
30. Lee IM, Rexrode KM, Cook NR, et al. Physical activity and coronary heart disease in women: is "no pain, no gain" passé? JAMA 2001;285(11):1447–54.
31. Bassuk SS, Manson JE. Physical activity and cardiovascular disease prevention in women: how much is good enough? Exerc Sport Sci Rev 2003;31(4):176–81.
32. Haskell WL, Lee IM, Pate RR, et al. Physical activity and public health: updated recommendation for adults from the American College of Sports Medicine and the American Heart Association. Circulation 2007;116(9):1081–93.
33. Eckel RH, Krauss RM. American Heart Association call to action: obesity as a major risk factor for coronary heart disease. AHA Nutrition Committee. Circulation 1998;97(21):2099–100.
34. Lewis CE, Jacobs DR Jr, McCreath H, et al. Weight gain continues in the 1990s: 10-year trends in weight and overweight from the CARDIA study. Coronary Artery Risk Development in Young Adults. Am J Epidemiol 2000;151(12):1172–81 B.
35. Kumanyika SK, Obarzanek E, Stettler N, et al. Population-based prevention of obesity: the need for comprehensive promotion of healthful eating, physical activity, and energy balance: a scientific statement from American Heart Association Council on epidemiology and prevention, interdisciplinary committee for prevention. Circulation 2008;118(4):428–64.
36. Berkel LA, Poston WS, Reeves RS, et al. Behavioral interventions for obesity. J Am Diet Assoc 2005;105(Suppl 1):S35–43.
37. Wadden TA, Butryn ML, Wilson C. Lifestyle modification for the management of obesity. Gastroenterology 2007;132(6):2226–38.
38. Wing RR. Behavioral approaches to the treatment of obesity. In: Bray GA, Bourchard C, James WPT, editors. Handbook of obesity: clinical applications. 2nd edition. New York: Marcel Dekker; 2004. p. 147–67.
39. Burke LE, Warziski M, Styn MA, et al. A randomized clinical trial of a standard versus vegetarian diet for weight loss: the impact of treatment preference. Int J Obes 2008;32:166–76.
40. Burke LE, Sereika SM, Music E, et al. Using instrumented paper diaries to document self-monitoring patterns in weight loss. Contemp Clin Trials 2008;29(2):182–93.
41. Baker RC, Kirschenbaum DS. Weight control during the holidays: highly consistent self-monitoring as a potentially useful coping mechanism. Health Psychol 1998;17(4):367–70.
42. Turk MW, Yang K, Hravnak M, et al. Randomized clinical trials of weight loss maintenance: a review. J Cardiovasc Nurs 2009;24(1):58–80.
43. National Institutes of Health Consensus Development Panel. Gastrointestinal surgery for severe obesity. Ann Intern Med 1991;115(12):956–61.
44. Mango VL, Frishman WH. Physiologic, psychologic, and metabolic consequences of bariatric surgery. Cardiol Rev 2006;14(5):232–7.
45. Buchwald H, Avidor Y, Braunwald E, et al. Bariatric surgery: a systematic review and meta-analysis. JAMA 2004;292(14):1724–37.
46. Sjostrom L, Lindroos A, Peltonen M, et al. Lifestyle, diabetes, and cardiovascular risk factors 10 years after bariatric surgery. N Engl J Med 2004;351(26):2683–753.
47. Schroetter SA, Peck SD. Women's risk of heart disease: promoting awareness and prevention—a primary care approach. Medsurg Nurs 2008;17(2):107–13.

48. Godtsfredsen NS, Osler M, Vestbo J, et al. Smoking reduction, smoking cessa-tion, and incidence of fatal and non-fatal myocardial infarction in Denmark 1976-1998: a pooled cohort study. J Epidemiol Community Health 2003;57: 412–6.
49. Kelley GA, Kelley KS. Aerobic exercise and HDL2-C: a meta-analysis of random-ized control trials. Atherosclerosis 2006;184:207–15.
50. Donnelly JE, Jacobsen DJ, Heelan KS, et al. The effects of 18 months of intermit-tent vs. continuous exercise on aerobic capacity, body weight and composition, and metabolic fitness in previously sedentary, moderately obese females. Int J Obes 2000;24(5):566–72.
51. Baigent C, Keech A, Kearney PM, et al. Efficacy and safety of cholesterol-lowering treatment: prospective meta-analysis of data from 90,056 participants in 14 randomised trials of statins. Lancet 2005;366(9493):1267–78.
52. Hamman RF, Wing RR, Edelstein SL, et al. Effect of weight loss with lifestyle inter-vention on risk of diabetes. Diabetes Care 2006;29(9):2102–7.
53. Ratner R, Goldberg R, Haffner S, et al. Impact of intensive lifestyle and metformin therapy on cardiovascular disease risk factors in the diabetes prevention program. Diabetes Care 2005;28(4):888–94.
54. Andajani-Sutjahjo S, Ball K, Warren N, et al. Perceived personal, social and envi-ronmental barriers to weight maintenance among young women: a community survey. Int J Behav Nutr Phys Act 2004;1(1):15–21.
55. Mosca L, Mochari H, Christian A, et al. National study of women's awareness, preventive action, and barriers to cardiovascular health. Circulation 2006; 113(4):525–34.
56. National Heart Lung and Blood Institute. North American Association for the study of obesity. Practical guide to the identification, evaluation, and treatment of overweight and obesity in adults. Available at: http://www.nhlbi.nih.gov/guidelines/obesity/ prctgd_c.pdf. Accessed February 26, 2009.

Genetics: Breast Cancer as an Exemplar

Rebekah Hamilton, PhD, RN

KEYWORDS

• Ethics • Genetics • Genomics • Nursing advocacy
• Nursing competencies

GENETICS OF HEREDITARY BREAST CANCER

The progress made in the discovery of disease-causing genes accelerated greatly with the initiation of the worldwide Human Genome Project in 1990.[1] While the number of tests for specific diseases continues to grow, one of the earliest presymptomatic mutation tests was for the disease of hereditary breast and ovarian cancer (HBOC). Breast cancer susceptibility gene 1 (BRCA1) and breast cancer susceptibility gene 2 (BRCA2) are the two major genes associated with HBOC.[2] The BRCA1 gene is located on chromosome 17 and the BRCA2 gene on chromosome 13.[3,4] Mutations in either of these genes significantly increase individuals' risk for breast and ovarian cancer across their lifespan (70 years), the mean cumulative cancer risks for mutation carriers being: breast cancer risk of 57% (95% confidence interval [CI], 47%–66%) for BRCA1 and 49% (95% CI, 40%–57%) for BRCA2 mutation carriers; and ovarian cancer risk of 40% (95% CI, 35%–46%) for BRCA1 and 18% (95% CI, 13%–23%) for BRCA2 mutation carriers.[5] Risks in identified carriers of either mutation are higher when based on other family members being diagnosed with breast cancer before the age of 35 years.[6]

Everyone has a BRCA1 and BRCA2 gene. These genes are tumor suppressor genes so that if a mutation occurs in such genes then the normal controls on cell growth are lost.[7] The mutations are passed down through generations in a dominant Mendelian pattern, meaning *each* offspring has a 50% chance of inheriting the parental mutation.[8] A genetic test is available to determine if a mutation is present in either gene.[9] It is recommended that a family member with breast or ovarian cancer be the first tested to determine if a mutation is present in the BRCA1 or BRCA2 gene.[10] If a mutation is identified in a family member then others who have not been diagnosed with breast or ovarian cancer can be tested to determine if they carry the mutation, and if they do then they too have an increased risk for cancer development.

The specter of breast cancer in HBOC families is significant. Research shows multiple cases of breast cancer across generations.[11,12] Women in these families can tell story after story of grandmothers, mothers, aunts, and cousins being

Funding support: NINR & NHGRI, 5R03NR009483-02.
Department of Women, Children and Family Health Science, College of Nursing, University of Illinois at Chicago, 845 South Damen Avenue, Chicago, IL 60612, USA
E-mail address: hamilr@uic.edu

diagnosed with breast cancer. One study participant from the author's research discussed how her mother had broken the "50 year" barrier:

> *Okay my mother is definitely the third generation to have breast cancer in her thirties. My grandmother had breast cancer at 38 and passed away. My mother is 51 now she is the first woman in our family to live past 50 in 5 generations.*

Many young women in HBOC families have experienced the loss of their own mothers, an event that only heightens the risk they feel for themselves:

> *Yeah, it's completely different... a lot of people worry about dying from the same things that their parents died from but I guess I have one up on that... it's more than just worrying about dying from what my mom died from it's like I have the genetic code and that makes it a really good possibility.*

Genetics is understood as being deterministic.[13] Women without a BRCA mutation overestimate their risk for developing breast cancer,[14–16] whereas those with a mutation express "inevitability" that if they do not make the difficult choices for prophylactic mastectomy or oophorectomy they will develop cancer.[17–19] Guidelines have been established to address the issue of genetic risk for breast cancer.

GUIDELINES FOR TESTING AND MANAGEMENT OF GENETIC RISK FOR BREAST CANCER

The National Comprehensive Cancer Network (NCCN) has established guidelines for testing for BRCA mutations and for the management of individuals who have a mutation in the BRCA1 or BRCA2 genes.[10] Genetic testing is recommended if an individual has one or more of the following familial characteristics:

- Early age (<50 years) onset of breast cancer (consider maternal and paternal sides independently)
- Two breast primaries or breast and ovarian cancer in a single individual or two breast primaries or breast and ovarian cancer in close relatives on the same side of the family
- Clustering of breast cancer with various other cancers such as male breast cancer, thyroid cancer, pancreatic cancer on the same side of the family
- Member of the family with a known BRCA mutation
- Member of a population at risk (eg, Ashkenazi Jewish)
- Male family member with breast cancer
- One or more cases of ovarian cancer on the same side of the family

It is recommended that any individual meeting one of the above criteria be referred to a professional genetic counselor for assessment. If the woman tests positive for one of the BRCA mutations, the NCCN[10] has published guidelines for health care providers that should be followed for these women:

Recommended management of individuals that have been identified as carrying a BRCA mutation includes the following:

- Self-breast examination monthly starting at age 18 years
- Clinical breast examination, semiannually, starting at age 25 years
- Annual mammogram and breast magnetic resonance imaging (MRI) starting at age 25 years or based on earliest age of onset in family
- Prophylactic oophorectomy between ages 35 and 40 years or on completion of childbearing

- For individuals not electing a prophylactic oophorectomy, concurrent transvaginal ultrasound, and CA125 levels semiannually starting at age 35 years or 5 to 10 years earlier than the first diagnosed case of ovarian cancer in the family
- Consider chemoprevention options (eg, tamoxifen)
- Consider research studies testing investigational imaging and screening options.

It is clear that such recommendations are meant to lower the woman's risk or identify a cancer as early as possible in the development of the disease.

RISK ACROSS THE LIFESPAN

One of the corresponding experiences of following these screening guidelines is that a woman is in frequent interaction with health care providers across her lifespan. If she is a young woman who has not received a breast cancer diagnosis, she faces the choice between breast and ovarian screening and a prophylactic mastectomy or prophylactic oophorectomy. It has been shown that a prophylactic oophorectomy reduces the risk of breast cancer in women with BRCA mutations by 50% or more.[19,20] The recommendation is that women have this surgery by the age of 40 years or when childbearing is completed.[10] Although the screening guidelines recommend the decision on a prophylactic mastectomy be considered by individual case, it has been shown that a prophylactic mastectomy reduces the risk of breast cancer in women with a BRCA1/2 mutation by approximately 90%.[21] Whereas mammography and breast MRI may identify breast cancer very early, the screening for ovarian cancer is much less efficient and not considered adequate for this at-risk population.[22] If a woman chooses to follow the screening guidelines but chooses against surgical interventions, she will interact with various health care providers at least four times each year, significantly more than a typical healthy young woman.

An aspect of having a genetic risk for a disease is that even when the disease is not present it affects the individual's life.[23-26] One result of this risk is that the "disease" is present across the lifespan of the woman. Even if a woman has no cancer diagnosis, she becomes a "patient," which can occur as young as age 18 years when as an adult she may choose to have the presymptomatic genetic test. The cumulative risk for breast cancer increases across the lifespan. For example, a 30-year-old woman with a BRCA1 mutation has a 3.2% risk, a 40-year-old with a BRCA1 mutation has a 19.1% risk, whereas a 70-year-old woman with BRCA1 reaches the cumulative risk of 85%.[27]

Research with young women (age 18–39 years)[11,23] has shown that for some women who have genetic testing for the BRCA mutation, life changes in that they cannot "undo" the knowledge they received. For some this is comforting; for example, this 32-year-old explained it this way:

I definitely have a feeling of gratitude that I live in a time where I can have this information to do with as I see fit, to reduce my risk or increase my surveillance or put my head in the sand—my mother and grandmother never had that alternative. Some women have made the analogy that knowing you carry a BRCA mutation is like having a "ticking time bomb" inside you—frankly, I would rather hear the ticking, be able to do what I could to prepare for the explosion, than just have it silently counting down, while I'm ignorant of its existence.

Others, however, do not find knowing easy to live with even if they do not question their decision to have the BRCA mutation genetic test:

For the last couple of years, or even several years, knowing about my genetic mutation has colored my general outlook on life. I do believe we all carry certain genetic mutations and that most diseases are probably genetically based, but knowing for certain that I have BRCA1 and that I have a very high risk of another breast cancer, or possibly other certain cancers, certainly "hangs" over my head in my daily life. I'm glad I was informed, because there are certain choices I can make and certain things I can do to closely monitor myself. At the same time, knowing this has made me more pessimistic regarding the opportunity for a long and healthy natural lifespan.

Kenen[25] introduced the idea of living with chronic risk to assess how individuals who had attended a high-risk breast cancer clinic in the United Kingdom but who do not know their mutation status. These participants used various coping strategies "to get on with their lives" but even not knowing if they carried a mutation, they found it difficult not to be concerned that they too might develop cancer. Living with the actual knowledge of genetic risk is a relatively new phenomenon. Whereas before the availability of presymptomatic genetic tests for diseases like breast cancer, individuals, such as those in Kenen's study[25] might have thought they had a higher risk because of their family history, the knowledge of an actual mutation seems to create a sense of inevitability of developing breast cancer. It was no longer a matter of "if" but "when" as one research participant described: "As I recall, I felt it was inevitable that I would die of breast cancer one day, and that played a part in how hopeless and awful I felt." The experience of daily living with BRCA genetic test results has not been well documented. Some studies report a sense of loneliness and social separation in individuals with BRCA mutations.[26,28] Others document the barriers to disclosing genetic test results to family.[29–32]

Most studies of the HBOC population that have used standardized measures of distress, anxiety, depression, and cancer worries support the emerging consensus that women who have a BRCA mutation do not experience major mental health risks.[33–37] It has been shown, however, that women who reported higher levels of distress at baseline continued to report higher distress as long as 6 months after receiving BRCA mutation test results.[37] A recent study comparing pretest psychological distress of women having the BRCA mutation testing with healthy controls showed that the high-risk women reported higher distress levels than the controls.[38] d'Agincourt[39] found in a qualitative study that a subset of her participants experienced a loss of agency after genetic testing and felt less control over their future health. The author's longitudinal study of women who know they carry a BRCA mutation but have not had a cancer diagnosis indicates a hypervigilance over a 4-year span, whereby the next screening examination could "be the one" that finds cancer.[40] Women who live with the knowledge of a BRCA mutation that significantly increases their risk of breast cancer do so in a new world of genetic health care and although research provides some information, the long-term consequences of having knowledge of genetic risk is still largely an uncharted domain.

BRCA TESTING AS AN EXEMPLAR FOR GENETIC HEALTH CARE

Four autosomal dominant cancers for which there is clinical presymptomatic genetic testing are HBOC; two forms of colon cancer, hereditary nonpolyposis colorectal cancer (HNPCC) and familial adenomatous polyposis (FAP), and multiple endocrine neoplasia.[41] Whereas all cancers have a genetic component, these four have been identified to have specific mutations that are inherited in families in a Mendelian dominant pattern. For the purpose of this article, the BRCA-associated breast cancer is used as an exemplar of genetic medicine. Quotations from research by Hamilton and colleagues with women who have a BRCA mutation[11,23,40,42] are used to illustrate the experience from the woman's perspective.

GENETICS IS FAMILIAL

It has been argued that "genetic information is different"[41,43] because of the nature of that information. First of all, genetics is familial. This fact means that whereas a woman, exercising her own autonomy, may decide to have a presymptomatic BRCA test, the knowledge she receives potentially impacts other family members whether or not they were consulted before the testing. Although most families do share genetic test results,[31,32,44] not all family members are willing participants in the genetic testing process. One research participant spoke of the differences with her sisters:

I think the way we've handled it in all the four sisters has been very, very different. Um, my sisters don't like to talk about it, don't want to deal with it, the two sisters that have chose not to be tested. And that's very difficult for me because I need to talk about this...and that's my way of coping. By their not dealing with it I definitely felt a sense of isolation and it, just pretending... like we have to pretend that somehow this is all OK when it's not.

Other investigators[45] have also found that in families genetic test participants often feel a strong sense of responsibility to inform immediate and extended family members of the potential risk they face. Women describe going to great lengths to contact aunts, uncles, and cousins: "So I found it really hard to, to make these contacts with all the family, to try to pull together the information and like it was a huge responsibility." Those who test first feel not only a responsibility to inform but to somehow set a standard as to how to deal with this information:

It sucks to be first. I feel like I always have to have the answers and be the voice of reason. So even though I'm a basket case to my sweet husband, to my brothers and sisters I feel like I have to be at peace with all of this. If I'm not, how can I expect them to be? I don't want them to live scared because of this.

Genetic information sets up many complex communications and interactions within families. Health care providers benefit from being aware of potential barriers as well as expectations faced by their patients.

GENES ARE "PASSED DOWN"

The definition of genetics implies the fact that what a parent has may be inherited by their offspring. This basic fact is important in understanding how individuals and families may react to information gained from genetic testing. Studies report the guilt parents feel when their daughters test positive for a BRCA mutation.[19,46,47] Younger women who are considering their reproductive choices also ponder and worry about the possibility of passing on the mutation, but only one of more than 80 research participants decided not to have children based on that issue alone (R.J. Hamilton, unpublished data, 2003.) Most participants acknowledge the risk but believe medicine will have found a cure by the time their offspring may face an actual cancer diagnosis:

As far as worrying about my (future) daughters carrying the mutation, I think breast cancer is something that has become more preventable and treatable, and is becoming even more so with advances in modern medicine. So I don't worry about that.

Although young women may not change their plans to have children, there is an acknowledgment that life is different because of the nature of a genetic risk for a specific disease:

My family is no longer as lighthearted as we once were. Genetic discussions happen all the time. I feel like there is absolutely no escaping this disease. And I know that the chances of having to watch someone I love go through this are high and that breaks my heart.

The sense that genetic risk will always be present adds to the burden some participants feel after genetic testing both for themselves and their offspring. Unlike other diseases that may have a contributing genetic component along with environmental influences, diseases such as HBOC cannot at this time be altered to any significant degree by health behavior choices. Whereas a smoker can stop smoking, an individual with a BRCA mutation may live a healthier lifestyle and shift the age of onset of breast cancer but not alter the actual risk of breast cancer development.[48] There is an "inescapability" component to HBOC that is described by women with the mutation:

It suddenly makes the possibility of cancer for the siblings—and their children— a real possibility. And with BRCA it is not just about breast cancer—but also ovarian cancer—and to a lesser extent other cancers like pancreatic cancer, prostate cancer. My two sisters all have sons so the latter is a factor. With BRCA, it just doesn't stop in the female line—it affects the males as well. A huge can of worms and worries was opened with my test results.

The very characteristic of genetics being something that is passed down through the generations creates varied and complex issues for families having such knowledge.

GENETICS AND DECISION MAKING

Usually through examining the family pedigree, individuals and family members may become aware that they potentially carry a BRCA mutation; these family members face many decisions. The first decision is whether to have the genetic test or not. If individuals choose to have the test and receive a positive result (eg, they have a mutation in the gene), then the follow-up decision is to increase screening or consider prophylactic surgery (see Guidelines Section). An individual who receives a positive BRCA mutation test knows that her risk of breast cancer onset is significantly higher than the general population.[5] Individuals may decide not to have the test. If this is the decision, depending on the woman's age she may find it more difficult to get insurance to pay for increased screening without a genetic test result. For example, a 30-year-old woman who decided not to have the test may not be covered for a mammogram because the recommended screening guidelines do not recommend mammograms before the age of 40 years.[49] Young women who are potentially at risk for carrying a BRCA mutation and choose not to be tested are unlikely to be offered early screening examinations. If the young woman does indeed have a BRCA mutation she risks not identifying a cancer early in its progression. If an individual has the test and tests negative for a known family mutation, her risk is the same as the general population. However, a significant proportion of women who have the genetic test receive what is called a variant of unknown clinical significance (VUCS). Such a change in the DNA may or may not represent deleterious mutation.[10,50] BRCA mutations account for only 20% to 25% of familial aggregation of breast cancers,[51] meaning most women who have testing will receive a VUCS result. Data from the Breast Cancer Information Core (http://research.nhgri.nih.gov/bci) estimates that 32% and 53% of all detected BRCA1 and BRCA2 mutations, respectively, are VUCS.[50] It is unclear whether this population has a risk equivalent to those with an identified mutation or equivalent to the general population. For this group, the NCCN[10] guidelines recommend offering these women opportunities to participate in research studies that work to identify risk associated with VUCS mutations or provide individualized recommendations based on family history. For example, if a woman's genetic test indicated a VUCS but she had a sister that developed breast cancer in her early 30s, then recommendations would be that the unaffected sister have intensive surveillance starting in her early to mid 20s.

Some research suggests that women who have had a breast cancer diagnosis but who test negative or VUCS doubt their results: "I often wonder if my cancer is still genetic—and that there are other markers besides BRCA 1 & 2—and could my type be worse?" A recent publication[52] indicated that women who receive VUCS and who entered the genetic testing process with a higher perceived risk of carrying a mutation continued to report higher levels of genetic testing distress over the course of a year. In an early study by Lerman and colleagues[53] 30% of women 25 to 39 years old who were not carriers of a BRCA mutation and had no breast cancer diagnosis continued to have follow-up mammograms 1 year after genetic testing. Because this group of women is not recommended to have mammograms until age 40, this activity suggests that they are not completely reassured by their negative BRCA test. Similar results have been reported with individuals who test negative for the FAP gene, which significantly increases risk for colorectal cancer.[54] It is unclear why a negative test result is not reassuring, although indications of the impact of family experiences with breast cancer suggest that women who have lived through the experience of multiple family members with breast cancer frame their risk perceptions on the family experience and not only the BRCA mutation test result.[11,36]

If a woman tests positive for a BRCA mutation she is then faced with decisions about surveillance or prophylactic surgery. The recommendation is for alternating mammogram and breast MRI and ovarian surveillance with CA125 levels and transvaginal ultrasound every 6 months. It has been reported that breast MRI is more sensitive but less specific than mammography, resulting in a higher false-positive rate leading to 3 times as many unneeded biopsies.[55] Women describe the difficulty of the experience of biopsies on suspicious findings on a MRI:

In addition to mammography, I have been given the option to have routine breast MRIs. There is a high rate of "false positives" or abnormal breast tissue anomalies which ultimately trigger additional biopsies. I have had three I think. This has been very challenging emotionally.

The other aspect of surveillance is the women's worry about being told at their next appointment that breast cancer has been identified:

It's almost like a time bomb.... I don't know when, but I'm pretty sure it will "go off" before I am age 40. It's the anxiety I feel each time I know I have an appointment coming up and wonder... will this be the time they find something?

Women describe not being able to live with this sense of anxiety over the next surveillance appointment and so they decide to go ahead with prophylactic surgeries:

More and more I would hear about young women in their late 20s and early 30s getting diagnosed with the cancer. I would think about the possibility of me being diagnosed as if it was going to happen that day or the next or in the next week.

Finally, in May 2005 I elected to get a prophylactic bilateral mastectomy and reconstruction (24-year-old BRCA1+).

Some women cannot tolerate the idea of having any cancer, so the prospect of "catching it early" as is the case with the intensive surveillance is simply not good enough:

However, when I got the BRCA+ result, and was truly faced with such a high risk of breast cancer, and since my sister already had it, I figured it was just a matter of time before I got breast cancer, so all of a sudden early detection wasn't good enough. I DO NOT want breast cancer and the best way to reduce my risk the most is to have preventive mastectomy, thus I am planning it for July/August of 2006 (about 1 year, 3 months after receiving my BRCA+ results)

The choice to have a prophylactic oophorectomy is an issue of great concern for younger women largely due to reproductive concerns, sexuality changes, and early onset of menopause.[11,56,57] Young women speak of a sense of urgency to make decisions about the timing of having children:

I feel very pressured to have children soon in fact my doctor has told me that I have to have a full hysterectomy and oophorectomy by the time I am 35. I plan on having children before then but I also feel very limited you know I don't feel like "oh I can't have children because I may pass on the gene" but I feel like, you know, I am 24 now, I am married, I feel like I should start having children soon but I don't know if I am ready for that.

While women at high risk report relief from the fear of ovarian cancer after a prophylactic oophorectomy, they also report concerns about loss of libido, body image changes, and dealing with early-onset menopause.[58,59] The choices women face after finding out they have a BRCA mutation are difficult, and involve multiple aspects of their lives and their families' lives.

SUMMARY

Women's health is and will continue to be in increasing numbers of ways affected by the advances in genetic health care. Not only are women most likely to be the keepers of health histories in families but they also tend to be the communicators of risk.[32,45,60] Because the BRCA mutations were among the earliest mutations identified in cancer risk assessment, women have also been pioneers in both genetic testing and decision making after genetic testing. In some ways the BRCA-affected population has been one large experimental group as researchers and health care providers discover what women want; what they need; how they react to knowledge of genetic risk; what procedures lower or eliminate the genetic risk; the aftermath, both psychological and physical, of choosing one procedure over another; and the impact on quality of life for the individual and her family. While knowledge continues to grow, only time will allow an examination of the long-term effects such as the physical sequelae of prophylactic surgeries in young women; the psychological impact on offspring of women identified with a mutation; the impact on family coherence and communication; and the interaction of this at-risk population with their health care providers.

Examining the experiences of women with a BRCA mutation provides a window onto considering issues that may arise with genetically based cancers that present in adulthood. At present, genetic testing for cancers for which individuals have a 50% risk of inheriting from a parent with the mutation include hereditary HNPCC and FAP, and multiple endocrine neoplasia. Similar issues such as disclosure of test results, psychological distress, and follow-up care after testing have been reported in the HNPCC population.[61–65] As more cancer and other disease type mutations are discovered, the knowledge gained from the BRCA population may assist health care providers in providing knowledgeable and sensitive care to patients.

Genetics is increasingly considered an essential science for all areas of health care.[66] Nurses must be knowledgeable of the science of genetics and have skills to engage patients who are in different stages of their encounters with genetic risk and follow-up. Beyond that, nurses must also understand the complexities that may arise for individuals and families when a genetic diagnosis occurs. Because the nature of genetics is familial, the idea that an individual is singular in her concerns does not apply in genetic health care. Fortunately, nursing has a strong commitment as a practice discipline to view a patient holistically, and this history of practice will serve nurses well in the evolving age of genetic health care.

REFERENCES

1. DOE/NIH. History of the human genome project. website. Available at: http://www.ornl.gov/hgmis. 2002. Accessed on January 26, 2003.
2. Wooster R, Weber BL. Breast and ovarian cancer. N Engl J Med 2003;348(23): 2339–47.
3. Miki Y, Swensen J, Shattuck-Eidens D, et al. A strong candidate for the breast cancer and ovarian cancer susceptibility gene BRCA1. Science 1994;266: 66–71.
4. Wooster R, Bignell G, Lancaster J, et al. Identification of the breast cancer susceptibility gene BRCA2. Nature 1995;378:789–92.
5. Chen S, Parmigiani G. Meta-analysis of BRCA1 and BRCA2 penetrance. J Clin Oncol 2007;25(11):1329–33.
6. Antoniou A, Pharoah PDP, Narod S, et al. Average risk of breast cancer and ovarian cancer associated with BRCA1 and BRCA2 mutations detected in case series unselected for family history: a combined analysis of 22 studies. Am J Hum Genet 2003;72:1117–30.
7. Venkitaraman AR. Cancer susceptibility and the functions of BRCA1 and BRCA2. Cellule 2002;108:171–82.
8. Loescher LJ, Whitesell L. The biology of cancer. In: Tranin AS, Masny A, Jenkins J, editors. Genetics in oncology practice: cancer risk assessment. Pittsburgh (PA): Oncology Nursing Society; 2003. p. 23–56.
9. Fries MH, Holt C, Carpenter I, et al. Guidelines for evaluation of patients at risk for inherited breast and ovarian cancer: recommendations of the Department of Defense Familial Breast/Ovarian Cancer Research Project. Mil Med 2002; 167(2):93–8.
10. National Comprehensive Cancer Network Inc. The NCCN Clinical Practice Guidelines in Oncology™ Genetic/familial high-risk assessment: breast and ovarian: clinical practice guidelines in oncology. National Comprehensive Cancer Network. To view the most recent and complete version of the NCCN Guidelines, go online to Available at: www.nccn.org. Accessed March 11, 2009.
11. Hamilton RJ, Williams JK, Bowers BJ, et al. Life trajectories, genetic testing, and risk reduction decisions in 18-39 year old women at risk for hereditary breast and ovarian cancer. J Genet Couns 2008;18(2):147–54.

12. Kenen R, Ardern-Jones A, Eles R. Family stories and the use of heuristics: women from suspected hereditary breast and ovarian (HBOC) families. Sociol Health Illn 2003;25(7):838–65.

13. Skirton H, Eiser C. Discovering and addressing the client's lay construct of genetic disease: an important aspect of genetic health care? Res Theory Nurs Pract 2003;17(4):339–52.

14. Blanchard D, Erblich J, Montgomery GH, et al. Read all about it: the over-representation of breast cancer in popular magazines. Prev Med 2002;35:343–8.

15. Dillard AJ, McCaul KD, Klein WMP. Resisting good news: reactions to breast cancer risk information. Health Commun 2006;19:115–23.

16. Katapodi MC, Lee KA, Facione NC, et al. Predictors of perceived breast cancer risk and the relation between perceived risk and breast cancer screening: a meta-analytic review. Prev Med 2004;38:388–402.

17. Lloyd S, Watson M, Waites B, et al. Familial breast cancer: a controlled study of risk perception, psychological morbidity and health beliefs in women attending genetic counseling. Br J Cancer 1996;74(3):482–7.

18. Press N, Fishman JR, Koenig BA. Collective fear, individualized risk: the social and cultural context of genetic testing for breast cancer. Nurs Ethics 2000;7(3): 237–49.

19. Kauff ND, Satagopan JM, Robson ME, et al. Risk-reducing salpingo-oophorectomy in women with a BRCA1 or BRCA2 mutation. N Engl J Med 2002;346(21): 1609–15.

20. Rebbeck TR, Lynch HT, Neuhausen S, et al. Prophylactic oophorectomy in carriers of BRCA1 and BRCA2 mutations. N Engl J Med 2002;346(21):1616–22.

21. Friebel TM, Domchek SM, Neuhausen SL, et al. Bilateral prophylactic oophorectomy and bilateral prophylactic mastectomy in a prospective cohort of unaffected BRCA1 and BRCA2 carriers. Clin Breast Cancer 2007;7(11):875–82.

22. Oei A, Massuger L, Bulten J, et al. Surveillance of women at high risk for hereditary ovarian cancer is inefficient. Br J Cancer 2006;94:814–9.

23. Hamilton RJ, Bowers BJ. The theory of genetic vulnerability: a Roy model exemplar. Nurs Sci Q 2007;20(3):254–65.

24. Tessaro I, Borstelmann N, Regan K, et al. Genetic testing for susceptibility to breast cancer: findings from women's focus groups. J Womens Health 1997; 6(3):317–27.

25. Kenen R, Ardern-Jones A, Eeles R. Living with chronic risk: healthy women with a family history of breast/ovarian cancer. Health Risk Soc 2003;5(3):315–31.

26. Hallowell N, Foster C, Eles R, et al. Accommodating risk: responses to BRCA1/2 genetic testing of women who have had cancer. Soc Sci Med 2004;59: 553–65.

27. Petrucelli N, Daly MB, Culver JO, et al. BRCA1 and BRCA2 Hereditary breast/ovarian cancer. June 19, 2007. Available at: http://www.ncbi.nlm.nih.gov/bookshelf/br.fcgi?book=gene&part=brca1. Accessed March 12, 2009.

28. Kenen R, Ardern-Jones A, Eeles R. "Social separation" among women under 40 years of age diagnosed with breast cancer and carrying a BRCA1 or BRCA2 mutation. J Genet Couns 2006;15(3):149–62.

29. Patenaude A. Parent child communication about hereditary disease risks. ELSI transactions from cancer to genomic medicine. Cleveland, Ohio, 2008.

30. Tercyak KP, Hughes C, Snyder C, et al. Parental communication of BRCA1/2 genetic test results to children. Patient Educ Couns 2001;42(3):213–24.

31. Forrest K, Simpson SA, Wilson BJ, et al. To tell or not to tell: barriers and facilitators in family communication about genetic risk. Clin Genet 2003;64:317–26.

32. Hamilton RJ, Bowers BJ, Williams JK. Disclosing genetic test results to family members. J Nurs Scholarsh 2005;37(1):18–24.
33. van Oostrom I, Meijers-Heijboer EJ, Lodder LN, et al. Long-term psychological impact of carrying a BRCA1/2 mutation and prophylactic surgery: a 5-year follow-up study. J Clin Oncol 2003;21(20):3867–74.
34. Claes E, Evers-Kiebooms G, Denayer L, et al. Predictive genetic testing for hereditary breast and ovarian cancer: psychological distress and illness representations 1 year following disclosure. J Genet Couns 2005;14(5):349–63.
35. Meiser B. Psychological impact of genetic testing for cancer susceptibility: an update of the literature. Psychooncology 2005;14:1060–74.
36. Mellon S, Gold R, Janisse J, et al. Risk perception and cancer worries in families at increased risk for familial breast/ovarian cancer. Psychooncology 2008;17:756–66.
37. Smith AW, Dougall AL, Posluszny DA, et al. Psychological distress and quality of life associated with genetic testing for breast cancer risk. Psychooncology 2008; 17:767–73.
38. Dorval M, Bouchard K, Maunsell E, et al. Health behaviors and psychological distress in women initiating BRCA1/2 genetic testing: comparison with control population. J Genet Couns 2008;17(4):314–26.
39. d'Agincourt-Canning L. A gift or a yoke? Women's and men's responses to genetic risk information from BRCA1 and BRCA2 testing. Clin Genet 2006;70: 462–72.
40. Hamilton RJ, Williams JK, Bowers B, et al. Living with genetic test results for hereditary breast and ovarian cancer. J Nurs Scholarsh, accepted for publication.
41. Jenkins J, Masny A. Why should oncology nurses be interested in genetics? In: Tranin AS, Masny A, Jenkins J, editors. Genetics in oncology practice. Pittsburgh (PA): Oncology Nursing Society; 2003. p. 1–12.
42. Douglas H, Hamilton RJ, Grubs RE. The effect of BRCA gene testing on family relationships: a thematic analysis of qualitative interviews. J Genet Couns 2009. pre-pub online.
43. Collins F. Shattuck lecture—medical and societal consequences of the human genome project. N Engl J Med 1999;341(1):28–37.
44. Clarke S, Butler K, Esplen M. The phases of disclosing BRCA1/2 genetic information to offspring. Psychooncology 2008;17(8):797–803.
45. Hallowell N, Foster C, Eeles R, et al. Balancing autonomy and responsibility: the ethics of generating and disclosing genetic information. J Med Ethics 2003;29(2): 74–91.
46. Hallowell N, Ardern-Jones A, Eeles R, et al. Guilt, blame and responsibility: men's understanding of their role in the transmission of BRCA1/2 mutations within their families. Sociol Health Illn 2006;28(7):969–88.
47. d'Agincourt-Canning L. Genetic testing for hereditary breast and ovarian cancer: responsibility and choice. Qual Health Res 2006;16(6):97–118.
48. King M-C, Marks JH, Mandell JB. Breast and ovarian cancer risks due to inherited mutations in BRCA1 and BRCA2. Science 2003;302(24):643–6.
49. USPTF. Screening for breast cancer, topic page. Available at: http://www.ahrq. gov/clinic/uspstf/uspsbrca.htm. Accessed March 10, 2009.
50. Van Dijk S, Van Asperen CJ, Jacobi CE, et al. Variants of uncertain clinical significance as a result of BRCA1/2 testing: impact of an ambiguous breast cancer risk message. Genet Test 2004;8(3):235–9.
51. Nathanson KL, Wooster R, Weber B. Breast cancer genetics: what we know and what we need to know. Nat Med 2001;7(5):552–6.

52. O'Neill SC, Rini C, Goldsmith RE, et al. Distress among women receiving uninformative BRCA1/2 results: 12-month outcomes. Psychooncology 2009. Online prepub.

53. Lerman C, Hughes C, Croyle RT, et al. Prophylactic surgery decisions and surveillance practices one year following BRCA1/2 testing. Prev Med 2000;31: 75–80.

54. Michie S, Smith JA, Senior V, et al. Understanding why negative genetic test results sometimes fail to reassure. Am J Med Genet 2003;119:340–7.

55. Kriege M, Brekelmans CTM, Boetes C, et al. Efficacy of MRI and mammography for breast cancer screening in women with familial or genetic predisposition. N Engl J Med 2004;351(5):427–37.

56. Hallowell N, Mackay J, Richards M, et al. High-risk premenopausal women's experiences of undergoing oophorectomy: a descriptive study. Genet Test 2004;8(2):148–56.

57. Friedman LC, Kramer RM. Reproductive issues for women with BRCA mutations. J Natl Cancer Inst Monogr 2005;34:83–6.

58. Fry A, Busby-Earle C, Rush R, et al. Prophylactic oophorectomy versus screening: psychosocial outcomes in women at increased risk of ovarian cancer. Psychooncology 2001;10:231–41.

59. Meiser B, Tiller K, Gleeson MA, et al. Psychological impact of prophylactic oophorectomy in women at increased risk for ovarian cancer. Psychooncology 2000;9:496–503.

60. Wilson BJ, Forrest K, van Teijlingen ER, et al. Family communication about genetic risk: the little that is known. Community Genet 2004;7:15–24.

61. Geirdal AO, Reichelt JG, Dahl AA, et al. Psychological distress in women at risk of hereditary breast/ovarian or HNPCC cancers in the absence of demonstrated mutations. Fam Cancer 2005;4:121–6.

62. Keller M, Jost R, Haunstetter CM, et al. Comprehensive genetic counseling for families at risk for HNPCC: impact on distress and perceptions. Genet Test 2002;6(4):291–302.

63. Mesters I, Ausems M, Eichhorn S, et al. Informing one's family about genetic testing for hereditary non-polyposis colorectal cancer (HNPCC): a retrospective exploratory study. Fam Cancer 2005;4:163–7.

64. van Oostrom I, Meijers-Heijboer H, Duivenvoorden HJ, et al. A prospective study of the impact of genetic susceptibility testing for BRCA1/2 or HNPCC on family relationships. Psychooncology 2007;16(4):320–8.

65. Peterson SK, Watts BG, Koehly LM, et al. How families communicate about HNPCC genetic testing: findings from a qualitative study. Am J Med Genet C Semin Med Genet 2003;119C:78–86.

66. Collins FS. The Human Genome Project and the future of medicine. Ann N Y Acad Sci 1999;882:42–55.

Computer-Mediated Patient Education: Opportunities and Challenges for Supporting Women with Ovarian Cancer

Phensiri Dumrongpakapakorn, MSN, RN[a],
Kathy Hopkins, MS, RN[a], Paula Sherwood, PhD, RN, CNRN[a],
Kristin Zorn, MD[b], Heidi Donovan, PhD, RN[a],*

KEYWORDS

• Patient education • Computer-based • Ovarian cancer
• Symptom management • Chronic illness

Patient education has been defined as "a combination of learning and motivation activities designed to educate patients and family members about disease states or procedures and appropriate methods for self-care" (CINAHL, 2009). Patient education is a critical element of quality cancer care, essential for optimizing health outcomes and improving self-management.[1] In particular, providing effective patient education has been recognized as a vital nursing role that has a meaningful impact on a patient's health and quality of life.[2] Unfortunately, as cancer treatment becomes more complex and pressures to reduce costs increase, it becomes more and more difficult to meet patients' educational needs. Not surprisingly, cancer patients continue to report a lack of adequate information regarding their illness, treatment, and supportive services.[3–5]

Data has clearly demonstrated that effective patient education requires more than the provision of information. Although studies have shown improvements in knowledge after information-focused interventions, few studies have demonstrated changes in patients' behaviors or improvements in self-management or quality-of-life

Funding: NIH/NINR R01 NR010735 (H.D.); NIH/NINR R21 NR009275 (H.D.); NIH/NINR 5T32NR008857 (K.H.).
[a] Department of Acute and Tertiary Care, University of Pittsburgh School of Nursing, 336 Victoria Building, 3500 Victoria Street, Pittsburgh, PA 15261, USA
[b] Department of Obstetrics, Gynecology, and Reproductive Services, Division of Gynecology, Magee Women's Hospital, University of Pittsburgh Medical Center, 300 Halket Street, Pittsburgh, PA 15213, USA
* Corresponding author.
E-mail address: donovanh@pitt.edu (H. Donovan).

outcomes.[6–8] The goal of patient education is to not only increase patient knowledge but to change behavior, such as improving use of self-care strategies, adherence to treatment recommendations, or communication with health care providers. These types of outcomes require educational activities that enhance learning and motivation for behavior change. The most successful cancer patient education programs have implemented interventions comprising evidence-based information along with cognitive reframing and problem-solving techniques.[9–12] Although combining patient education with strategies to affect behavioral change has proven effective in improving patient outcomes, these interventions often require multiple time-intensive nurse-patient interactions that may be impractical or unrealistic in the current health care climate.[13]

Meeting the comprehensive needs of women with ovarian cancer can be especially challenging for clinicians. The vast majority of women are diagnosed at advanced stages, when the chances of a cure are unlikely.[14,15] Primary surgery and chemotherapy are often effective initially, but up to 80% of women ultimately experience a recurrence.[15,16] Following recurrence, women receive second-, third-, and "subsequent"-line therapies in an attempt to keep the cancer under control. In a study of 279 women with recurrent ovarian cancer, women had received an average of four different chemotherapeutic regimens,[17] resulting in multiple symptoms and side effects. On average, women with recurrent ovarian cancer experience 10 to 12 concurrent disease- and treatment-related symptoms, and higher numbers of concurrent symptoms have been associated with lower quality of life.[18–20] Effective symptom management education is essential to reduce negative outcomes in this patient population.

Patient education about managing multiple symptoms can be complex, requiring patients to learn, integrate, and apply a large amount of information. There is evidence that efforts to accomplish this within the constraints of a typical clinic appointment can be overwhelming to ovarian cancer patients and clinicians. Up to 40% of patients do not discuss even their most bothersome symptoms during their clinic visit, and up to 50% do not recall receiving recommendations for managing their most bothersome symptoms.[17]

Computers and Internet-based technologies have the potential to facilitate cost-effective delivery of symptom management interventions outside the traditional clinical setting. Each patient could process information at her own pace, review resources, reflect on recommendations, and work on program-specific recommendations. Computer-mediated symptom management education could take place at the patient's convenience without time pressures and the constraints of scheduling.

The purpose of this article is to review research studies of computer-mediated patient education interventions in persons with cancer or other chronic diseases to identify (1) common components of interventions, (2) evidence for the relative efficacy of different components, and (3) other factors associated with improved outcomes following computer-mediated patient education. Findings are discussed with respect to supporting women with ovarian cancer and specifically to the development and testing of WRITE Symptoms, a web-based symptom management program for women with recurrent ovarian cancer.

SEARCH STRATEGY

Three of the authors (P.D., K.H., and H.D.) conducted an initial literature search on PubMed using the following search strategy: (1) patient education (MeSH [Medical Subject Heading] or keyword) or health education (MeSH or keyword) or psychoeducation (keyword) = 98,323 results; (2) computer-based (key word) or computer-assisted instruction (MeSH or keyword) or telemedicine (MeSH or keyword) or internet

(MeSH or keyword) or internet-based (keyword) or web-based (keyword) = 48,405 results; (3) combined 1 and 2 = 3542 results; (4) limited 3 to randomized controlled trials (RCT) = 289. The following inclusion criteria were used to ensure relevance to the topic:

1. Patient education consisted of learning and motivation activities. Studies evaluating the effect of only information, social support, neurocognitive exercises, or telemonitoring with medication adjustment were excluded.
2. The patient education intervention required patient interaction or activity in response to computer-generated education, or computer-mediated educational interactions with a trained interventionist. Examples include responding to questions, practicing skills, or problem solving. Studies of read-only/view-only education modules were excluded.
3. Educational programs targeted patients with cancer or chronic disease. Chronic disease was defined as an illness of long duration that could be controlled but not cured. Studies targeting primary prevention, cancer screening, smoking cessation, weight loss, and alcohol misuse were excluded. Chronic disease was included because of the low number of articles focusing on cancer. In addition, patients with cancer and patients with chronic illnesses must all learn to develop a lifelong focus on managing the illness, associated symptoms, and the impact of those symptoms on their lives.
4. Programs that were limited to a single symptom (eg, insomnia or headache) or required a fundamentally different educational focus (eg, schizophrenia, eating disorders, infertility) than cancer disease and symptom management were excluded.

Of the 289 articles, 29 randomized clinical trials met these criteria. To ensure that the search strategy captured all relevant articles, all references of eligible articles were reviewed and a search was conducted for articles that cited the eligible study. Through this process several key articles were found that were not identified in the original search, therefore a second broader search was conducted using the following criteria: computer-assisted instruction (MeSH or keyword) or computer-assisted therapy (MeSH or keyword) or internet (MeSH or keyword) or telemedicine (MeSH or keyword) or computer-based (keyword) or internet-based (keyword) or web-based (key word). From 774 identified articles, 11 unique articles were discovered that met the same inclusion/exclusion criteria. In total, 40 randomized clinical trials of computer-mediated patient education for patients with cancer or chronic diseases were included in this review. The most common target populations for these studies were patients with diabetes (n = 18) and depression (n = 6). Three studies included patients with cancer.

FINDINGS
Common Components of Computer-Mediated Patient Education Interventions

Common components of interventions in the identified studies included provision of information, cognitive-behavioral approaches, skills training, peer support, expert advice, and communication training. Information was provided regarding the disease itself, associated symptoms, recommended treatments, or management strategies. Cognitive-behavioral approaches included formal cognitive-behavioral therapy (CBT), as well as other theoretically guided components designed to enhance adoption of new behaviors. Common components in this category included goal setting, problem solving, motivational interviewing, overcoming barriers, cognitive reframing, and self-management counseling. Skills training included practical "how to" information such as tips and skills for preparing nutritious foods, proper blood sugar monitoring techniques, and instructions on how to do relaxation or strengthening exercises. Peer support was another common component and included a variety of computer/Internet tools to connect patients suffering from the same illness. Specific tools included chat rooms, discussion boards, e-mail systems, and peer coaching. Many studies included access to a health care expert as part of their intervention; this access ranged from providing as-needed responses to patient-generated questions to conducting formal educational/counseling sessions at prescribed intervals. In some cases, computer-mediated activities with experts were supplemented by telephone or personal contacts. Finally, several interventions specifically focused on improving patient-health care provider communication through self-advocacy or communication training. **Table 1** provides a summary of the different categories of intervention components used in each of the reviewed studies. Information provision was the most common intervention component, followed by access to an expert and teaching cognitive-behavioral strategies.

Effectiveness of Computer-Mediated Patient Education Interventions

A wide range of outcomes were evaluated in the reviewed studies. For ease of synthesis, these outcomes were categorized as changes in: (1) knowledge and beliefs, (2) self-care behaviors, (3) social support, (4) patient health, and (5) health care use. Assessments of knowledge and beliefs included whether the patient retained provided information as well as the effect of interventions on concepts such as self-efficacy, barriers to change, and confidence. Measures of self-care behaviors were most common in studies of patients with diabetes and typically focused on assessments of dietary intake and physical activity. Other self-care behaviors that were measured included the use of stress management strategies and health care provider communication. Measures of patient health included physical and emotional outcomes and varied by target population. Studies of diabetes focused on hemoglobin A1c (HbA1c), body mass index (BMI; calculated as the weight in kilograms divided by height in meters squared), and cholesterol; depression studies focused on depression, anxiety, and functional outcomes; other studies included outcomes such as blood pressure, physical symptoms (pain and fatigue), disease-related distress, and quality of life. Few studies included assessments of perceived social support and health care outcomes. **Table 1** includes a summary of the number of each type of outcomes that were assessed as well as the number of outcomes that were significantly improved in each of the studies. Health care use as an outcome is not included in the table, but is discussed in the following sections. Overall, computer-mediated interventions have been shown to be effective in improving both physical and mental health outcomes in persons with chronic health conditions, particularly when an expert interventionist is used. Exemplars of successful studies highlighting intervention components and delivery methods that were effective are provided in the following sections.

Diabetes

In diabetes, Shea[25] and Glasgow and colleagues[30–33,36,37] evaluated two different approaches to computer-mediated patient education. To test the "Informatics for Diabetes and Education Telemedicine" (IDEATel) intervention, Shea recruited 1665 Medicare recipients with diabetes, aged 55 years or older, and living in federally designated medically underserved areas of New York. More than 75% of patients did not know how to use a computer and 93% reported a median income of less than $20,000. Patients assigned to the intervention were provided with computers and telemedicine units in their homes and participated in a range of activities that included: (1) videoconferencing between patients and a nurse case manager; (2) remote glucose monitoring with electronic upload and integration with the patient's electronic medical record; (3) access to a web portal that contained their own clinical data and secure web-based messaging with nurse case managers; and (4) access to an educational web site created for the project (regular and low literacy versions). One year post intervention, participants in the IDEATel intervention had significantly greater reductions in HbA1c, blood pressure, total cholesterol, and low-density lipoprotein cholesterol than those in the control group, who received standard care. Effects were strongest for participants who had HbA1c levels greater than 7 at baseline.

The investigators noted that Medicare claims were higher in the intervention group compared with the control group, an issue that warrants further exploration. It was hypothesized that providing patients in medically underserved areas with access to nurse case managers may have provided patients with the advice and encouragement to seek necessary care that they had not previously been receiving. A particular strength of this project was the focus on an underserved patient population and the provision of computers to patients with no previous computer experience. The findings provide important support for the generalizability of computer-mediated interventions, demonstrating that older, low-income patients without computer experience are willing to use and can benefit from computer-mediated education and disease management.

The work of Glasgow and colleagues is noteworthy for the investigators' efforts to create cost-effective studies that are highly generalizable. These researchers at the Oregon Research Institute (ORI) have developed a series of "practical clinical trials." Practical clinical trials are designed with clinically relevant interventions as control conditions, include a diverse patient population (broad study inclusion criteria), and recruit from heterogeneous practice settings.[61] The ORI studies have emphasized interventions that could move quickly to widespread adoption by virtue of being brief, fitting into the realities of clinic visits, and reducing demands on physicians.[32]

Glasgow and colleagues began their computer-mediated diabetes education programs in 1997 with an intervention that included 2 parts. The first was a brief (5- to 10-minute) computer-based assessment and feedback on dietary patterns, key barriers for dietary self-management, and preferences for self-care strategies. Two printouts were generated, one for the patient that focused on problem situations to plan for in dietary management, and an assessment summary for the physician. The second part of the intervention was a 20-minute session with a research interventionist who assisted with patient-centered goal setting and problem solving with self-help materials. Participants repeated the program at their 3-month follow-up visit and received telephone reinforcements at 1 and 3 weeks and 6 months post baseline. At 1 year post randomization, patients receiving the intervention had greater reduction in cholesterol and calories from fat, but no difference in HbA1c or BMI compared with the control group, who received computerized assessment and standard medical care only. Costs were estimated at $137 per participant with an estimate of $8 per mg/dl reduction in serum cholesterol. The investigators argued that these costs are low compared with pharmacologic interventions.

Over the past decade, Glasgow and colleagues have compared other iterations of their diabetes self-management program, moving it out of the office setting to a web-based delivery system that helps patients complete a self-directed diabetes program providing self-management information, automated goal setting, and problem solving. In 2003, the group published results of a three-arm trial (basic web-based program versus web-based program + peer support versus web-based

Table 1
Intervention components included in computer-mediated patient education interventions and outcomes assessed and improved as a result of interventions

Author, Year	Peer	Info	CBT	Skills	Expert	Comm	Belief A	Belief I	Behav A	Behav I	Social A	Social I	Health A	Health I	Total A	Total I
Diabetes																
Smith and Weinert, 2000[21] n = 30	X	X			X						1	0	2	0	3	0
Gerber et al, 2005[22] n = 244		X	X	X			3	1	1	0			4	0	8	1
Kim and Kang, 2006[23,a] n = 73		X	X	X	X				1	1			2	2	3	3
Jansa et al, 2006[24,b] n = 40		X			X		1	0	1	0			4	0	6	0
Shea, 2007[25,c] n = 1665		X			X +								5	5	5	5
Grant et al, 2008[26,d] n = 244		X				X							3	0	4	1
Wangberg, 2008[27] n = 64		X	X	X			1	0	1	1			1	1	2	1
Quinn et al, 2008[28] n = 30		X			X				4	3			1	1	5	4
Ralston et al, 2009[29] n = 83		X	X	X	X								5	2	5	2
Glasgow et al (Oregon Research Institute) Series																
Glasgow et al, 1997[30] n = 206		X	X		X				1	1			3	1	4	2
Glasgow and Toobert, 2000[31,e] n = 320		X	X		X+TFU				3	1			3	0	6	1
		X+CR	X		X				3	0			3	0	6	0
The Diabetes priority program (n = 886)																
Glasgow et al, 2004[32]		X	X		X				2	2			2	0	4	2
Glasgow et al, 2005[33]		X	X		X				1	1			4	0	5	1
Williams et al, 2007[34]		X	X		X		2	2							2	2
D-Net Program																
McKay, 2001[62] n = 78	X	X			X		1	0	1	0			1	0	2	0

Study																
Barrera et al, 2002[35,f]	X	X		X	X				2	2		2	2		2	2
n = 160	X	X		X	X				2	0		2	0		2	0
Glasgow et al, 2003[36,g]	X			X	X		1	0	4	0	2	1	7	0	14	1
n = 320	X			X	X		1	0	4	1	2	0	7	0	14	1
Tailored Self-Management Program (TSM)																
Glasgow et al, 2006[37,h]	X			X	X			2		1		1	5	1	7	2
n = 335																
Depression																
Clarke et al, 2002[38,i] n = 299	X			X						1		1	1	0	1	0
Clarke et al, 2005[39,j] n = 255	X			X						2		2	2	1	2	1
Andersson et al, 2005[40] n = 117	X	X		X					4	3		4	4	3	4	3
Beating the Blues (BtB) Program																
Proudfoot et al, 2003[42] n = 167	X	X		X					3			3	3	3	3	3
Proudfoot et al, 2004[43] and McCrone et al, 2004[44,k] n = 274	X	X		X					3			3	3	3	3	3
Chronic illness (unspecified)																
Lorig et al, 2006[46] n = 958	X			X			1	1	4	1		7	7	4	11	5
Hill et al, 2006[47] n = 120 (prelim analysis)	X			X			3	2	2		2	1	2	0	7	3
Weinert et al, 2008[48] n = 176	X			X			1	1	1	0			2		2	1
Leveille, 2009[41,l] n = 241			X		X		1	0					5	0	6	0
Cancer																
Gustafson et al, 2001[49,m] n = 246	X			X	X		2	0	3	2	3	3	4	0	12	5

(continued on next page)

Table 1
(continued)

Author, Year	Intervention Components						Dependent Variables									
							Belief		Behav		Social		Health		Total	
	Peer	Info	CBT	Skills	Expert	Comm	A	I	A	I	A	I	A	I	A	I
Davison and Degner, 2002[50] n = 749						X	1	0							1	0
Owen et al, 2005[51,n] n = 62	X	X	X										6	0	6	0
Cerebrovascular																
Southard et al, 2003[52] n = 104	X	X			X				2	0			11	2	13	2
Kwon et al, 2004[53] n = 110		X		X	X								7	1	7	1
Johnson et al, 2006[54] n = 1227		X	X						2	2					2	2
Green et al, 2008[55,o] n = 778																
Web		X		X			1	0	3	1			5	1	9	2
Web + Pharmacist		X	X	X	X		1	0	3	2			5	3	9	5
Arthritis																
Van den Berg et al, 2006[56] n = 160	X	X	X	X	X		1	1	1	1			3	0	4	1
Lorig et al, 2008[57] n = 885	X	X	X	X		X	1	1	7	2			8	4	16	7
Human immunodeficiency virus																
Flatley-Brennan, 1998[58,p] n = 57	X	X			X		2	0			1	1[I]	1	0	4	1[I]
Chronic pain																
Buhr-man et al, 2004[59] n = 56		X	X	X			1	0	8	3			5	0	14	3
Chronic obstructive pulmonary disease																
Nguyen et al, 2008[60,q] n = 50		X		X	X		1	0					4	0	5	0

Abbreviations: Intervention components: CBT, cognitive-behavioral techniques; Comm, communication training; Expert, clinician advice or coaching; Info, disease/treatment information; Peer, peer support; Skills, skill training. Dependent variables: A, assessed; Beliefs, knowledge/attitudes/beliefs; Behav, behavior; Health, health outcomes; I, improved as result of intervention; social, Social support.

[a] Three-arm trial, web-based (WB) and telephone nurse support versus printed material (PM) and telephone nurse support versus usual care (UC). Both WB and PM >> UC for all three outcomes. WB = PM. Key issue may be whether the telephone support was essential.

[b] Control condition in this trial is 12 face-to-face interactions. No significant differences between conditions. Both groups showed improvements in beliefs, behavior, and three of four health outcomes. Computer intervention is more cost-effective than face-to-face.

[c] Telemedicine with: (1) videoconferencing allowing patients to interact with nurse case managers; (2) remote monitoring glucose with electronic upload and integration with the electronic medical record; (3) access to secure web-based messaging with nurse case managers; (4) access to an educational web site created for the project (regular and low literacy versions) improved all targeted clinical outcomes at 1 year. Computers and telemedicine units were provided to subjects. Supports proposition that patients without computer experience can use these without difficulty.

[d] Good baseline control of HbA1c may have affected outcomes. Trend for group differences in improvements when looking at subset of patients with HbA1c >7 at baseline.

[e] Control condition in this trial is the previously tested intervention in Glasgow et al[30]. Adding telephone follow-up (TFU) or community resources (CR) did not improve outcomes more than the brief computerized intervention. All three groups showed improvements in fat intake, weight, and lipids. No significant impact on hemoglobin A1c (HbA1c) or quality of life.

[f] Control group was a web-based information and automated goal recommendation program. Peer support improved perceptions of social support.

[g] Although there were no significant differences between groups in this trial, the control group was a web-based diabetes information and automated target goal recommendation program. All three groups showed significant baseline to 10-month improvements on 11 of 14 outcomes, leading to the conclusion that the basic program is effective and that neither peer support nor tailored self-management coaching added to the benefits of the program.

[h] Employed "practical" clinical trial design to enhance representativeness and external validity but may have reduced ability to detect between-group differences.

[i] High rates of attrition and overall very low usage of site (median 2 sessions). Subgroup analyses showed intervention effect for those with mild depression (Center for Epidemiologic Studies Depression Scale <16) at 16 and 32 weeks.

[j] Same intervention as Clark et al[38] + postcard or telephone reminders to use program. Improved outcomes. In this follow-up study, subgroup analyses showed greater improvements in depression for the group who had higher depression at baseline.

[k] McCrone article describes health care use/cost-effectiveness outcomes of the study: 4 of 4 assessed cost-utility/effectiveness, improved lost hours from work.

[l] Nurse e-coaching focused solely on teaching patients to communicate more effectively—did not improve outcomes.

[m] Underserved population derived greatest benefit from the intervention.

[n] Broad inclusion criteria and relatively high functioning of subjects at baseline may have limited findings. Those with poorer perceived health status at baseline showed greater treatment effects than those with better perceived health.

[o] Addition of pharmacist-led education and planning significantly improved number and strength of outcomes.

[p] Social isolation was reduced through the intervention after controlling for depression. Importance of assessing and controlling for depression in these types of interventions. Communication features (e-mail and public bulletin board) were the most used and valued features.

[q] Control group was an established face-to-face dyspnea management program. Although there were no significant between-group differences, both web and face-to-face programs showed significant improvement on all five outcomes at 3 and 6 months.

program + expert self-management coaching) in which all three groups showed significant baseline to 10-month improvements on 11 of 14 outcomes. These investigators concluded that the basic program is effective and that neither peer support nor tailored self-management coaching added to the benefits of the program. However, without the use of a control group, it is impossible to know whether changes are a result of the web-based intervention or of other factors.

Depression

Proudfoot and colleagues[42–44] have developed and tested the Beat the Blues (BtB) web-based CBT program for depression. BtB is an 8-session self-help treatment program designed to be used by patients with no previous computer experience. Patients work through cognitive modules that help them to identify and challenge automatic thoughts that are counterproductive. Other modules focus on learning and practicing new behaviors such as activity scheduling, goal setting and problem solving, task breakdown, or sleep management. A final module helps the patient to work on action planning and relapse prevention. BtB includes a variety of approaches to engage users: interactive modules, animations and voice-overs, and filmed case studies of fictional patients to model CBT. Although interaction with a clinician is not an explicit part of the program, it is designed to facilitate interactions by providing a printed summary of the patient's work to the clinician at the end of each session. Proudfoot and colleagues[42,43] reported significant improvements in depression, anxiety, and work and social adjustment at 1-, 3-, and 6-month follow-up compared with control patients receiving standard care as prescribed by their general practitioner. BtB was also found to be cost-effective in terms of cost per quality-adjusted life year and lost employment costs.[44] As a result of this work, the BtB program is now considered the standard of care for those with mild to moderate depression in the United Kingdom.[45] At the time of diagnosis, general practitioners can provide patients with free access to the BtB online program.

Other chronic illnesses

Lorig and colleagues[46,57] have conducted a series of studies that progressed from establishing the efficacy of face-to-face self-management programs for persons with chronic illness, to developing web-based programs using a similar model, to extending the program to different patient populations. The program includes content to help participants design individualized exercise programs; cognitive symptom management such as relaxation, visualization, distraction, and self talk; methods for managing negative emotions such as anger, fear, depression, and frustration; an overview of medications; strategies for improving patient-provider communication; healthy eating; fatigue management; action planning; feedback; and methods for solving problems that result from living with a chronic disease. Over 6 weeks, participants are asked to log on at least three times a week for a total of 1 to 2 hours and to participate in the activities for that week. Participants are asked to do several activities including reading the week's content on web pages, posting an action plan on the bulletin board, checking in with a buddy via e-mail, and participating in self-tests and activities. The participants can post problems for discussion on the bulletin board, which invites responses from other members of the group as well as health care moderators. Lorig and colleagues reported that at 1-year follow-up, participants in the intervention group had significantly greater improvements in health-related distress, pain, fatigue, and shortness of breath compared with those in the control group receiving standard care.[46]

Cancer

Gustafson and colleagues[49] at the University of Wisconsin were pioneers in the use of computers to enhance the care of patients with cancer. In 2001, they developed and tested the Comprehensive Health Enhancement Support System (CHESS) for women diagnosed with breast cancer. The web-based CHESS intervention was comprised "Information Services" (answers to frequently asked questions; full articles on breast cancer; consumer guide to health services; referral directory to services); "Support Services" (peer discussion groups, Ask an Expert, and personal stories of how others facing breast cancer coped); and "Decision Services" (assessment of a person's emotional status followed by coping advice; system for recording and tracking health changes; decision aid to learn about options, clarify values and understand consequences of choices; and goal setting and action planning). In this study, 246 women were randomly assigned to CHESS versus care as usual (supplemented with Susan Love's Breast Book). Participants in CHESS were given 6 months of access to the web site. At 2 and 5 months follow-up, the study participants in CHESS scored significantly higher in social support and information competence than the control group. There were no significant differences between groups in four quality-of-life outcomes including social/family well-being, emotional well-being, functional well-being, and breast cancer concerns.[49] The investigators also reported significant interactions based on race, education, and lack of insurance such that women of color, those with less education, and those without insurance saw greater improvements as a result of CHESS in social support, information support, and participation in health care.

In summary, the use of theoretically guided components to enhance adoption of new behaviors (eg, CBT, problem solving, self-management, and counseling) seemed to improve multiple patient outcomes. In depression, computer-based CBT alone improved depression as long as efforts were included to ensure subjects used the site. For chronic diseases in which complex management or medication adjustment is necessary (eg, diabetes, hypertension, CAD, cancer), expert medical advice or coaching was critical; few studies showed improved outcomes without providing contact with a trained expert.

Few studies evaluated mechanisms underlying intervention effects. Those that did identified level of engagement in the intervention (those who used it more had better outcomes) as a predictor of improved outcomes.[62] In addition, self-efficacy seemed to be an important predictor of intervention effects. Patients who started with higher levels of self-efficacy or showed greater improvements in self-efficacy over time tended to have better outcomes.[46] Those who were at increased risk for negative outcomes (eg, poorly controlled blood sugar, poorly managed hypertension) also tended to have more benefit.[26,51] Finally, vulnerable patient populations (minorities, elderly, and those with low incomes) seemed to gain the most benefit from computer-mediated patient education programs.[25,48]

A common critique of internet-based health intervention research is that noncomputer-literate users will not be able to participate. The findings from this review are counter to this critique. Other reviews of the use of computer-mediated interventions have found them to be feasible and acceptable to patients/subjects in a wide variety of clinical populations, using a variety of technologies.[63,64] In an early and compelling call to ensure universal access to health information and support, Eng and colleagues[65] argued that there are substantial data to show that members of underserved groups desire and will use health information technology, and that when barriers to access are removed and training is provided, underserved populations (including the elderly, residents of inner cities and rural areas, and racial and ethnic minorities) can all successfully use technology.

Development of a Computer-Mediated Symptom Management Program for Women with Recurrent Ovarian Cancer: WRITE Symptoms

Findings from this review suggest that computer-mediated interventions could be developed to support women with ovarian cancer. Results also provide important information on necessary intervention components as well as study design considerations. Based on these findings and the specific symptom management needs of women with ovarian cancer, Donovan and colleagues developed WRITE Symptoms (Written Representational Intervention To Ease Symptoms). WRITE Symptoms is a computer-mediated intervention that builds on effective components of previous symptom management and computer-mediated interventions. WRITE Symptoms is based on the Representational Approach to patient education, a seven-element intervention aimed at facilitating conceptual change, which includes a comprehensive assessment of patient representations; explorations of gaps, concerns, or misconceptions; provision of evidence-based symptom management recommendations; assistance with goal setting and problem solving; and follow-up and reevaluation.[66,67]

In its first iteration, WRITE Symptoms was tested as a web-based delivery system through which patients were able to interact with a research nurse over their own private message boards. Using asynchronous postings, nurses led each patient through the WRITE Symptoms intervention to develop individualized goals and strategies for improving symptom management. A pilot study of 65 women with recurrent ovarian cancer supported that the nurse-delivered WRITE Symptoms is a feasible, acceptable intervention, with preliminary evidence supporting baseline to 5- and 9-week improvements in symptom representation (severity, distress, and consequences).[18]

A key question is whether individualization by nurses is critical to the success of the WRITE Symptoms Intervention, or whether women can be guided through the program by a web-based, interactive computer module without assistance from a nurse (referred to as "Self-directed WRITE Symptoms"). In the second phase of intervention development, a web-based computer module was developed that leads patients through the same theoretical components as the nurse-delivered WRITE Symptoms intervention: guiding women through a self-assessment of their health problems, providing information on common concerns that women face when trying to manage multiple and complex symptoms, providing evidence-based recommendations for symptom management, and guiding patients through a process of developing individualized goals and strategies to improve symptom management.

A three-arm RCT is currently underway, funded by the National Institute of Nursing Research (R01 NR010735NINR) and supported as a Gynecologic Oncology Group Protocol (GOG-259), to compare the efficacy of these two different web-based delivery systems (nurse-delivered via private web-based message boards versus self-directed using a web-based computer module) versus usual care in a sample of 480 women with recurrent cancer recruited from Gynecologic Oncology Group sites across the United States. Primary outcomes are symptom representation (severity, distress, consequences) and quality of life. By carefully examining critical components of WRITE Symptoms, the mechanisms through which it is effective, and for which individuals it is most effective, this study has the potential to advance the science of computer-mediated patient interventions and enhance cancer symptom management across diverse patient populations.

REFERENCES

1. Gosselin TK. Patient education is essential in providing quality cancer care. ONS News 1999;14(12):1.

2. Suter PM, Suter WN. Patient education. Timeless principles of learning: a solid foundation for enhancing chronic disease self-management. Home Healthc Nurse 2008; 26(2):82–8 [quiz 89–90].

3. Hordern A, Street A. Issues of intimacy and sexuality in the face of cancer: the patient perspective. Cancer Nurs 2007;30(6):E11–8.

4. Steele R, Fitch MI. Supportive care needs of women with gynecologic cancer. Cancer Nurs 2008;31(4):284–91.

5. Thompson HS, Littles M, Jacob S, et al. Posttreatment breast cancer surveillance and follow-up care experiences of breast cancer survivors of African descent: an exploratory qualitative study. Cancer Nurs 2006;29(6):478–87.

6. Craddock RB, Adams PF, Usui WM, et al. An intervention to increase use and effectiveness of self-care measures for breast cancer chemotherapy patients. Cancer Nurs 1999;22(4):312–9.

7. Dodd MJ. Efficacy of proactive information on self-care in chemotherapy patients. Patient Educ Couns 1988;11(3):215–25.

8. Williams SA, Schreier AM. The effect of education in managing side effects in women receiving chemotherapy for treatment of breast cancer. Oncol Nurs Forum 2004;31(1):E16–23, Online.

9. Given B, Given CW, McCorkle R, et al. Pain and fatigue management: results of a nursing randomized clinical trial. Oncol Nurs Forum 2002;29(6):949–56, Online.

10. Given C, Given B, Rahbar M, et al. Does a symptom management intervention affect depression among cancer patients: results from a clinical trial. Psychoon-cology 2004;13(11):818–30.

11. Rawl SM, Given BA, Given CW, et al. Intervention to improve psychological functioning for newly diagnosed patients with cancer. Oncol Nurs Forum 2002;29(6): 967–75, Online.

12. Sherwood P, Given BA, Given CW, et al. A cognitive behavioral intervention for symptom management in patients with advanced cancer. Oncol Nurs Forum 2005;32(6):1190–8, Online.

13. Keulers BJ, Welters CF, Spauwen PH, et al. Can face-to-face patient education be replaced by computer-based patient education? A randomised trial. Patient Educ Couns 2007;67(1–2):176–82.

14. Bhoola S, Hoskins WJ. Diagnosis and management of epithelial ovarian cancer. Obstet Gynecol 2006;107(6):1399–410.

15. Gadducci A, Cosio S, Zola P, et al. Surveillance procedures for patients treated for epithelial ovarian cancer: a review of the literature. Int J Gynecol Cancer 2007;17(1):21–31.

16. Hauspy J, Covens A. Cytoreductive surgery for recurrent ovarian cancer. Curr Opin Obstet Gynecol 2007;19(1):15–21.

17. Donovan HS, Hartenbach EM, Method MW. Patient-provider communication and perceived control for women experiencing multiple symptoms associated with ovarian cancer. Gynecol Oncol 2005;99(2):404–11.

18. Donovan HS, Ward S, Sherwood P, et al. Evaluation of the Symptom Representation Questionnaire (SRQ) for assessing cancer-related symptoms. J Pain Symptom Manage 2008;35(3):242–57.

19. Portenoy R, Thaler H, Kornblith A, et al. Symptom prevalence, characteristics and distress in a cancer population. Qual Life Res 1994;3(3):183–9.

20. Wenzel LB, Donnelly JP, Fowler JM, et al. Resilience, reflection, and residual stress in ovarian cancer survivorship: a gynecologic oncology group study. Psy-chooncology 2002;11(2):142–53.

21. Smith L, Weinert C. Telecommunication support for rural women with diabetes. Diabetes Educ 2000;26(4):645–55.
22. Gerber BS, Brodsky IG, Lawless KA, et al. Implementation and evaluation of a low-literacy diabetes education computer multimedia application. Diabetes Care 2005;28(7):1574–80.
23. Kim C-J, Kang D-H. Utility of a Web-based intervention for individuals with type 2 diabetes: the impact on physical activity levels and glycemic control. Comput Inform Nurs 2006;24(6):337–45.
24. Jansa M, Vidal M, Viaplana J, et al. Telecare in a structured therapeutic education programme addressed to patients with type 1 diabetes and poor metabolic control. Diabetes Res Clin Pract 2006;74(1):26–32.
25. Shea S. The Informatics for Diabetes and Education Telemedicine (IDEATel) project. Trans Am Clin Climatol Assoc 2007;118:289–304.
26. Grant RW, Wald JS, Schnipper JL, et al. Practice-linked online personal health records for type 2 diabetes mellitus: a randomized controlled trial. Arch Intern Med 2008;168(16):1776–82.
27. Wangberg SC. An internet-based diabetes self-care intervention tailored to self-efficacy. Health Educ Res 2008;23(1):170–9.
28. Quinn CC, Clough SS, Minor JM, et al. WellDoc mobile diabetes management randomized controlled trial: change in clinical and behavioral outcomes and patient and physician satisfaction. Diabetes Technol Ther 2008;10(3):160–8.
29. Ralston JD, Hirsch IB, Hoath J, et al. Web-based collaborative care for type 2 diabetes: a pilot randomized trial. Diabetes Care 2009;32(2):234–9.
30. Glasgow RE, La Chance P-A, Toobert DJ, et al. Long term effects and costs of brief behavioural dietary intervention for patients with diabetes delivered from the medical office. Patient Educ Couns 1997;32(3):175–84.
31. Glasgow RE, Toobert DJ. Brief, computer-assisted diabetes dietary self-management counseling: effects on behavior, physiologic outcomes, and quality of life. Med Care 2000;38(11):1062–73.
32. Glasgow RE, Nutting PA, King DK, et al. A practical randomized trial to improve diabetes care. J Gen Intern Med 2004;19(12):1167–74.
33. Glasgow RE, Nutting PA, King DK, et al. Randomized effectiveness trial of a computer-assisted intervention to improve diabetes care. Diabetes Care 2005;28(1):33–9.
34. Williams GC, Lynch M, Glasgow RE. Computer-assisted intervention improves patient-centered diabetes care by increasing autonomy support. Health Psychol 2007;26(6):728–34.
35. Barrera M Jr, Glasgow RE, McKay H, et al. Do internet-based support interventions change perceptions of social support? an experimental trial of approaches for supporting diabetes self-management. Am J Community Psychol 2002;30(5):637–54.
36. Glasgow RE, Boles SM, McKay H, et al. The D-Net diabetes self-management program: long-term implementation, outcomes, and generalization results. Prev Med 2003;36(4):410–9.
37. Glasgow RE, Nutting PA, Toobert DJ, et al. Effects of a brief computer-assisted diabetes self-management intervention on dietary, biological and quality-of-life outcomes. Chronic Illn 2006;2(1):27–38.
38. Clarke G, Reid E, Eubanks D, et al. Overcoming Depression on the Internet (ODIN): a randomized controlled trial of an internet depression skills intervention program. J Med Internet Res 2002;4(3):E14.

39. Clarke G, Eubanks D, Kelleher C, et al. Overcoming depression on the internet (ODIN) (2): a randomized trial of a self-help depression skills program with reminders. J Med Internet Res 2005;7(2):e16.
40. Andersson G, Bergstrom J, Hollandare F, et al. Internet-based self-help for depression: randomised controlled trial. Br J Psychiatry 2005;187(5):456–61.
41. Leveille SG, Huang A, Tsai SB, et al. Health coaching via an internet portal for primary care patients with chronic conditions: a randomized controlled trial. Med Care 2009;47(1):41–7.
42. Proudfoot J, Goldberg D, Mann A, et al. Computerized, interactive, multimedia cognitive-behavioural program for anxiety and depression in general practice. Psychol Med 2003;33(2):217–27.
43. Proudfoot J, Ryden C, Everitt B, et al. Clinical efficacy of computerised cognitive-behavioural therapy for anxiety and depression in primary care: randomised controlled trial. Br J Psychiatry 2004;185:46–54.
44. McCrone P, Knapp M, Proudfoot J, et al. Cost-effectiveness of computerised cognitive-behavioural therapy for anxiety and depression in primary care: randomised controlled trial. Br J Psychiatry 2004;185:55–62.
45. National Institute for Health and Clinical Excellence (NICE). Computerised cognitive behaviour therapy for depression and anxiety. London (UK): National Institute for Health and Clinical Excellence; 2006. No. 97.
46. Lorig KR, Ritter PL, Laurent DD, et al. Internet-based chronic disease self-management: a randomized trial. Med Care 2006;44(11):964–71.
47. Hill W, Weinert C, Cudney S. Influence of a computer intervention on the psychological status of chronically ill rural women: preliminary results. Nurs Res 2006; 55(1):34–42.
48. Weinert C, Cudney S, Hill W. Health knowledge acquisition by rural women with chronic health conditions: a tale of two web approaches. Aust J Rural Health 2008;16(5):302–7.
49. Gustafson DH, Hawkins R, Pingree S, et al. Effect of computer support on younger women with breast cancer. J Gen Intern Med 2001;16(7):435–45.
50. Davison BJ, Degner LF. Feasibility of using a computer-assisted intervention to enhance the way women with breast cancer communicate with their physicians. Cancer Nurs 2002;25(6):417–24.
51. Owen JE, Klapow JC, Roth DL, et al. Randomized pilot of a self-guided internet coping group for women with early-stage breast cancer. Ann Behav Med 2005; 30(1):54–64.
52. Southard BH, Southard DR, Nuckolls J. Clinical trial of an internet-based case management system for secondary prevention of heart disease. J Cardiopulm Rehabil 2003;23(5):341–8.
53. Kwon H-S, Cho J-H, Kim H-S, et al. Establishment of blood glucose monitoring system using the internet [see comment]. Diabetes Care 2004;27(2):478–83.
54. Johnson SS, Driskell M-M, Johnson JL, et al. Efficacy of a transtheoretical model-based expert system for antihypertensive adherence. Dis Manag 2006;9(5): 291–301.
55. Green BB, Cook AJ, Ralston JD, et al. Effectiveness of home blood pressure monitoring, Web communication, and pharmacist care on hypertension control: a randomized controlled trial. JAMA 2008;299(24):2857–67.
56. van den Berg MH, Ronday HK, Peeters AJ, et al. Using internet technology to deliver a home-based physical activity intervention for patients with rheumatoid arthritis: a randomized controlled trial. Arthritis Rheum 2006;55(6):935–45.

57. Lorig KR, Ritter PL, Laurent DD, et al. The internet-based arthritis self-management program: a one-year randomized trial for patients with arthritis or fibromyalgia. Arthritis Rheum 2008;59(7):1009–17.
58. Flatley-Brennan P. Computer network home care demonstration: a randomized trial in persons living with AIDS. Comput Biol Med 1998;28(5):489–508.
59. Buhrman M, Faltenhag S, Strom L, et al. Controlled trial of internet-based treatment with telephone support for chronic back pain. Pain 2004;111(3):368–77.
60. Nguyen HQ, Donesky-Cuenco D, Wolpin S, et al. Randomized controlled trial of an internet-based versus face-to-face dyspnea self-management program for patients with chronic obstructive pulmonary disease: pilot study. J Med Internet Res 2008;10(2):e9.
61. Tunis SR, Stryer DB, Clancy CM. Practical clinical trials: increasing the value of clinical research for decision making in clinical and health policy. JAMA 2003; 290(12):1624–32.
62. McKay HG, King D, Eakin EG, et al. The diabetes network internet-based physical activity intervention: a randomized pilot study. Diabetes Care 2001;24(8): 1328–34.
63. Krishna S, Balas A, Spencer DC, et al. Clinical trials of interactive computerized patient education: implications for family practice. J Fam Pract 1997;45(1):25–33.
64. Murray E, Burns J, See TS, et al. Interactive health communication applications for people with chronic disease. Cochrane Database Syst Rev 2005;(4): CD004274.
65. Eng TR, Maxfield A, Patrick K, et al. Access to health information and support: a public highway or a private road? JAMA 1998;280(15):1371–5.
66. Donovan HS, Ward S. A representational approach to patient education. J Nurs Scholarsh 2001;33(3):211–6.
67. Donovan HS, Ward SE, Song M-K, et al. An update on the representational approach to patient education. J Nurs Scholarsh 2007;39(3):259–65.

Women's Mental Health: Depression and Anxiety

Robynn Zender, MS*, Ellen Olshansky, DNSc, WHNP-BC, FAAN

KEYWORDS

- Women • Mental health • Anxiety • Depression
- Co-morbid conditions

Mental disorders affect about one in four adults annually, or 57.7 million people when applied to the 2004 United States census population, and are the leading cause of disability in the United States and Canada for persons aged 15 to 44 years.[1] The Global Burden of Disease study revealed that mental illness, including suicide, accounts for greater than 15% of the burden of disease in established market economies, which is more than the disease burden caused by all cancers.[1] Many people suffer from concurrent mental disorders, with nearly half meeting the criteria for two or more disorders. The severity of a mental disorder is strongly related to comorbidity (the presence [or effect] of one or more disorders or diseases in addition to [or upon] a primary disease or disorder), meaning that a disorder is often more severe if comorbid conditions exist.[1] Depression and anxiety often present together and are examples of such comorbid conditions.[1-3] About one-half of those with a primary diagnosis of major depression also have an anxiety disorder. This comorbidity is so pronounced that some investigators have theorized these disorders as stemming from similar causes.[3]

But what is unique about women's mental health? Gender. Sex ratios for selected mental disorders such as major depressive disorder, anxiety disorder, posttraumatic stress disorder, seasonal affective disorder, and eating disorders are much higher in women than men.[4] Women are more likely than men to have severe depressions and to relapse, with biologic differences in hormone profiles affecting mental health disorder risks and symptoms, the course of those disorders, and recovery.[3-5] The female to male ratio of depression at puberty rises from 1:1 to 2:1, pointing to estrogen and progesterone and their known influences on brain function and stress response as culprits.[4] Women also exhibit an increased vulnerability to depression during times of reproductive endocrine change such as in premenstrual, postpartum, and perimenopausal periods.[1,4] Sex-based differences in the size and structure of the human brain, with men having larger brains and women having lighter, more complex brains and

Program in Nursing Science, College of Health Sciences, University of California, 233 Irvine Hall, Irvine, CA 92697, USA
* Corresponding author.
E-mail address: rzender@uci.edu (R. Zender).

proportionately larger frontal lobes (which function in socialization, judgment, memory, and language), may also contribute to the differential presentation in women.[4]

In 1 year, about 7% of Americans will suffer a mood disorder, with unipolar major depression ranking first in causes of disability worldwide.[3] Women between the ages of 18 and 45 comprise the majority of those with major depression.[3] Anxiety disorders are the most prevalent mental disorder in adults, and affect twice as many women as men.[3] In the United States, 1-year prevalence rates for all anxiety disorders among adults aged 18 to 54 years exceeds 16%, and there is significant comorbidity with mood and substance abuse disorders.[3]

The cause of mood and anxiety disorders is not precisely known, but may be triggered by stressful life events and enduring stressful social conditions, and are affected by biologic, genetic, and psychosocial factors such as brain chemistry, hormonal balance, socioeconomic status, support network, diet, premorbid medical conditions, cognition, personality, and gender.[3]

In addition to depression and anxiety existing comorbidly and along with other mental disorders, mental disorders have common comorbidity with somatic illness, including diabetes mellitus, human immunodeficiency virus/AIDS,[6] ischemic heart disease, stroke, cancer, chronic lung disease, arthritis, Alzheimer disease, and Parkinson disease.[3] Although other mental disorders exist, this article focuses on depression and anxiety in women, and other conditions comorbid with depression or anxiety: cardiac disease, obesity, vitamin D deficiency, and irritable bowel syndrome.

DEPRESSION

Depression is the most common mental illness experienced by women.[7] The lifetime prevalence of depression in women is about 21% compared with 13% in men, and it is the second leading cause of disease burden for women in the United States,[2] with rates on the rise:[2,7] women today have a 10 times greater chance of suffering from depression than their grandmothers did.[2] The risk of depression increases as women age,[3] and anxiety symptoms are present in about 58% of depressed outpatients.[2] The course of depression across the life span is marked by recurrent episodes of depressive symptoms followed by periods of remission, and the course of depression tends to be more chronic in late life than in younger adults.[3] For some, an initial episode of major depression will evolve over time (with remissions and recurrences) into unipolar major depression, whereby each new episode confers new and more severe risks of chronicity, disability, and suicide.[3] Major depression is associated with considerable impairment in functioning, comparable to and sometimes worse than that experienced by patients suffering from a variety of chronic medical conditions.[7] One study reported that depressed outpatients function at lower levels than outpatients with any other illness except cardiac illness.[5]

Depression has many forms including major depressive disorder, dysthymic disorder, psychotic depression, postpartum depression, and seasonal affective disorder, and is characterized by persistent sadness, anxiousness, hopelessness, guilt, worthlessness, irritability, restlessness, loss of interest in activities or hobbies, fatigue, difficulty concentrating, impaired memory and decision making, insomnia or hypersomnia, overeating or appetite loss, suicidal ideation or attempts, or persistent aches or pains, headaches, cramps, or digestive problems that do not ease with treatment.[1] Symptoms interfere with normal functioning in daily life, and persist for a matter of months to years.[1] Ten to fifteen percent of patients formerly hospitalized with depression commit suicide, with major depressive disorder accounting for 20% to 35% of all deaths by suicide.[3]

The greatest risk factor for a future depressive episode is a past depressive history.[2] Women who have a history of depression are nearly five times more likely to have a future episode of major depressive disorder, with the risk of recurrence increasing with each episode, and an association with a stressful life event becoming progressively weaker with each new depressive episode.[2]

Treatment of depression most often includes pharmacologic agents in conjunction with cognitive-behavioral therapy or interpersonal therapy, the combination proving important for full recovery and preventing relapses.[2] However, an even more aggressive and comprehensive program that includes dietary and lifestyle changes including regular exercise and sleep, a diet high in w-3 fatty acids, tryptophan, folic acid, vitamin D, and vitamin B complex, exposure to bright light, spiritual "therapy," and complementary and alternative medicines like acupuncture, may bring about even more thorough and long-lasting recovery.[8,9]

ANXIETY

Anxiety disorders, the most frequently occurring mental disorders, are diagnosed twice as often in women, and encompass a group of conditions that share extreme or pathologic anxiety as the principal disturbance of mood or emotional tone.[3] Categories of anxiety disorder include generalized anxiety disorder, panic disorder, agoraphobia, specific phobia, social phobia, obsessive-compulsive disorder, acute distress disorder, and posttraumatic stress disorder.[3] Presentation of anxiety disorders, in general, include a surge in heart rate, sweating, tensing of muscles, worry, easy fatigability, poor memory or concentration, insomnia, irritability, compulsive behaviors, dissociation, and somatic symptoms.[3] What the myriad of anxiety disorders have in common is a state of increased arousal or fear, often occurring with no immediately recognizable external stressor.[3] Anxiety is often characterized as "the extreme of normal fear,"[3,10] although some investigators theorize that anxiety is born of a different process than a continuum of severity.[10] Anxiety disorders often have an early age of onset, are chronic, have high rates of relapse and recurrence, and the rate of comorbid anxiety in suicide is likely underestimated. Panic disorder and agoraphobia, in particular, are associated with an increased risk of attempted suicide.[3]

Anxiety disorders are strongly and independently associated with chronic medical illness, low levels of physical health-related quality of life, and physical disability.[6] Various anxiety disorders have shown greater association than depression with 4 chronic physical disorders, namely hypertension, arthritis, asthma, and ulcers, and convincing evidence exists that anxiety is associated with high rates of medically unexplained symptoms and increased use of health care resources.[6]

Similar to depression, treatment often consists of a combination of medications and psychotherapy.[1] Outcomes are also likely to be improved if dietary and lifestyle changes are incorporated into one's daily agenda.[1]

DEPRESSION AND ANXIETY IN CHILDHOOD AND ADOLESCENCE

Mood disorders are one of the most impairing classes of emotional and behavioral disturbances in youth, causing problems in social, academic, and interpersonal functioning.[11] Depressive symptoms are normative in children and adolescents, with most of these populations reporting depressive symptoms at some point before adulthood.[11] Nondiagnostic levels of depressive symptoms occur at high rates, with point prevalence estimates ranging from 20% to 30% in adolescents.[11] Before puberty, boys and girls are equally likely to develop depressive disorders but by age 15 years, girls are twice as likely as boys to have experienced a major depressive disorder.[1,11]

Diagnosis-level depressive disorders have a point prevalence of 2.8% for children younger than 13 years and 5.6% for 14- to 18-year-olds.[11] Children aged 8 years and younger show rates of less than 1%.[11] Depression in childhood often persists, recurs, and continues into adulthood, especially if untreated, and is a strong predictor of more severe illness in adulthood.[1]

As with the adult population, anxiety is the most common co-occurring disorder with mood disorders in adolescents, primarily panic and generalized anxiety disorder, with a lifetime prevalence of anxiety of up to 75% in depressed adolescents.[11] Other commonly occurring comorbid conditions with childhood depression are disruptive behavior disorders, such as conduct disorder and attention-deficit/hyperactivity disorder (14%–36%), and substance abuse (45%–50%).[11] Depression in children also has several common occurring somatic complaints, such as sleep difficulties, appetite and subsequent weight changes, headaches, chronic back or chest pain, gastrointestinal difficulties, decreased libido in adolescents, generalized complaints of not feeling well, aching extremities, excessive fatigue, and dizziness.[11]

Whereas diagnostic criteria are the same for children as adults, depressive symptoms can present differently in children. For example, with major depressive disorder in children, disruptiveness may be more easily expressed than internal emotions, so that internalized problems such as depression may be overlooked, with attention focused on the outward behavior.[11] Irritability may also present more commonly than depressed mood or sadness in children. Children often use language to reveal inner thought processes, such as feelings of worthlessness, and a negative view of the world and of the future.[11] The most commonly displayed emotions by depressed children are irritability, indifference, lack of cooperation, and disinterest.[11]

Although anxiety disorders are one of the most prevalent categories of pediatric psychopathology,[12] classifying the disease process of anxiety is controversial; some investigators theorize the disorder as existing on a continuum of normal fear whereas others propose that anxiety represents a different neurologic process altogether.[10] Diagnosis of anxiety in childhood and adolescence is controversial too, due to disagreement over what constitutes normal versus pathologic childhood behavior, difficulty in assessing distress in children, and lack of clear, empirically valid diagnostic criteria.[10]

Childhood prevalence studies of being diagnosed with any anxiety disorder report that 3-month estimates range from 2.2% to 8.6% and 6-month estimates range from 5.5% to 17.7%.[12] When ascertained retrospectively, lifetime prevalence rates reportedly range from 8.3% to 27%.[12] In youth diagnosed with generalized anxiety disorder (GAD), more than one associated symptom is usually endorsed (although only one associated symptom of restlessness, fatigue, difficulty concentrating, irritability, muscle aches or tension, or sleep difficulties is required for diagnosis), with restlessness the most common and muscle tension the least common.[12] Because of high comorbidity rates of generalized anxiety disorder with depression, it is speculated as to whether the two are distinct disorders.[12] The terms "sequential comorbidity" and "cumulative comorbidity" have been used to describe the relationship between the two disorders, depending on whether they occur one after the other (usually GAD being diagnosed first),[11] or occur during a lifetime but not in a simultaneous manner.[12]

Although little is known about the antecedents and determinants of childhood anxiety disorders, the etiology of depression in children is often approached from a biopsychosocial framework.[11,12] Treatment for both disorders is often a combination of medications and psychotherapy, which have shown substantial progress in recent years.[10–12]

Nurses are often the first line of medical contact for children, whether in school or a primary care setting. By understanding how depression and anxiety present differently in children and adolescents behaviorally, cognitively/verbally, and with somatic symptoms, a nurse may decrease the amount of time between a child presenting with a complaint and receiving proper diagnosis and treatment of the problem.[11,12]

MENSTRUATION-, PREGNANCY-, AND MENOPAUSE-RELATED DEPRESSION AND ANXIETY

Premenstrual syndrome (PMS) is a medically unexplained disorder that presents with physical, psychological, and behavioral symptoms during the luteal phase of the menstrual cycle and typically resolves after the onset of menstruation.[13] Mild symptoms are common, occurring in approximately 75% of women of reproductive age,[13] with clinical prevalence of PMS between 19% and 30%,[14] and up to 8% of women experiencing a form of PMS extreme enough to severely disrupt normal functioning, possibly resulting in suicidal ideation or attempt.[13] This most severe variant of PMS is termed premenstrual dysphoric disorder, which presents with at least one mood symptom (typically low mood, tension, anger, irritability, or mood swings) and suffering physical or psychological symptoms in most menstrual cycles in the past year.[15,16] The most frequently reported symptoms of PMS are irritability, depression, fatigue, water retention, weight gain, breast tenderness, headaches, abdominal cramps, and mood swings.[17]

Severe PMS symptoms most commonly appear in the late second decade of life, and may be associated with a history of major depressive disorder and anxiety disorders.[17] In a 2007 study, symptom reporting for PMS was related to depression among women exposed to cigarette smoke, reflecting the strong correlation between cigarette smoking and lifetime prevalence of depression.[17] In a perimenopausal cohort, PMS symptoms were reported by 26% of depressed women compared with only 9% of nondepressed women.[17] Increasing age has been associated with a decreased reporting of premenstrual anxiety, whereas caffeine intake shows a positive association with premenstrual anxiety.[17]

Current treatment relies primarily on self-management, dietary modifications including vitamin supplementation, exercise, stress management, and cognitive-behavioral therapies. Women who are unable to adequately control symptoms through lifestyle changes may benefit from prescription medications.[15,16]

Ante-, peri-, and postpartum depression occur in 10% to 20% of women, with rates of depression increasing in the last 2 trimesters of pregnancy up to 51% in the general population of pregnant women.[18] Women are at greater risk of developing depression in the postpartum period than at any other time in the life cycle,[19] and postpartum depression is considered the most common postdelivery complication of childbirth.[20,21] Women with postpartum depression may be greater than four times as likely to screen positive for depression 4 years later than controls who were not depressed postpartum.[20] Postpartum depression may affect the mother's physical health,[18–20] the physical and emotional health of the offspring,[18–21] and that of family members.[3,19] Antenatal predictors of postpartum depression include antenatal depression (a 6.5-fold increase in risk)[18] or anxiety, previous infertility,[22] past history of psychiatric illness, lack of social support, and stressful life events.[20]

Depression occurs in about 20% and up to 50% of pregnant women,[18] with women particularly vulnerable to depression and anxiety if they have high-risk pregnancies or are put on bed rest.[23] Women with antenatal depression are less likely to attend regular prenatal visits, follow prenatal advice, including taking supplements, and are more likely to engage in fetal abuse (such as physical assault by punching the pregnant abdomen, or engaging in risk behaviors like tobacco, alcohol, or drug use).[18] Stress and depression increase maternal serum corticosteroid and catecholamine levels, which are suspected of decreasing placental blood flow, which may in turn induce fetal stress and cause fetal brain and heart rate changes.[18] Depression has been positively associated with increased uterine irritability, pregnancy-induced hypertension, preeclampsia, antepartum bleeding, decreased uterine artery blood flow, preterm delivery, increased planned cesarean section, and epidural anesthesia.[18] Babies of depressed mothers are at higher risk of lower Apgar scores, less breastfeeding, failure to thrive, and increased admissions to neonatal intensive care.[18]

Although it is important to screen high-risk women for depression before, during, and after pregnancy, the high prevalence and deleterious effects of depression provide strong evidence for universal screening.[18,19] In screening for postpartum depression, when contact with the health care system might afford the best results in terms of identifying and responding to health needs, "crucial" moments have been proposed as at 6 hours, 6 days, 6 weeks, and 6 months postdelivery, loosely interpreted.[19] Nursing care, including home visits, enjoys a strong position in the assessment and detection of depression, education of coping skills, and referrals to appropriate adjunct health care workers to remediate depressive symptoms and their consequences.[19]

As in pregnancy, the menopausal transition is a natural life event that is sometimes marked by depression and anxiety. Whereas anxiety disorders in the general United States population have about a 26% prevalence, that prevalence is higher in women and increases significantly in women, but not in men, at midlife (after age 45), with reports of anxiety, stress, and tension common during menopause.[14] Persistent anxiety has been shown to increase during the menopausal transition independently of depressive symptoms.[14] A vulnerability to anxiety symptoms was found in naturally menopausal women who had premenstrual syndrome (2 times greater risk of anxiety), high perceived stress (40% greater), and a history of depression (2 times greater).[14] Greater anxiety symptoms have also been reported in women with early bilateral oophorectomy, sexual dysfunction, and lapses in physical activity in the early postmenopausal period, and have been strongly linked with both number and severity of hot flushes.[14]

Regarding depression during menopause, many theories have been developed and tested over the years, and there remains a controversy.[24–26] The research clearly shows that most women do not develop depression as they transition into menopause; however, in a subset of women an increased risk for developing major and minor depressions during the menopausal transition exists.[24] Although menopause has been identified as an independent risk factor for depression at midlife, a past history of depression, whether related to reproductive endocrine change or not (ie, postpartum depression) may[26] or may not[24] predict the onset of depression during the menopausal transition. A growing body of evidence suggests that the risk of clinical depression and depressive symptoms increases during the perimenopause in relation to hormonal changes, but then decreases in the postmenopausal period.[14,25] Depression in women around the time of menopause is seen most often, and with greater severity, in the 2 or 3 years before menstruation stops.[25] The latest research indicates that developing depression during the menopausal transition contains pieces of a continuum of risk (history of postpartum depression, previous stressful events) and evidence of a critical window of vulnerability during this time of life (menopause-related sleep problems, vasomotor symptoms, and health indicators).[26]

Treatment of depression in menopause most often includes antidepressant medication, psychotherapy, or a combination of the two, similar to the treatment of depression in other periods of life.[24] However, a recent study suggests the use of high-dose estrogen in the treatment of "the triad of hormone-responsive depressive disorders," meaning when premenstrual depression, postpartum depression, and depression in the years leading up to menopause occurs in the same vulnerable women.[25] The recommended dose for perimenopausal, but not postmenopausal, depression is transdermal estrogen patches of 200 µg.[25]

DEPRESSION AND ANXIETY COMORBIDITY WITH SOMATIC ILLNESS

Cardiovascular disease (CVD) has been the leading cause of mortality in the United States for over 100 years, with one in three American adults now dying from one or more types of CVD, accounting for 1 out of every 2.8 deaths in 2004 and more deaths each year than cancer, chronic lung disease, accidents, and diabetes mellitus combined.[6] Risk factors for CVD that are modifiable include hypertension, diabetes mellitus, hypercholesterolemia, elevated body mass index, unhealthy diet, and sedentary lifestyle. Chronic stress, depression, and anxiety also increase the risk of developing CVD and complicate recovery following acute cardiac events.[6]

Depression has long been noted in occurrence with CVD and cardiac death, but the association has been validated scientifically only in the last 15 years or so.[27] Major depression in hospitalized patients with coronary artery disease have reported prevalence of between 17 % and 27%,[27] and is both a risk factor for incident CVD and a predictor of poor outcome in cardiac patients.[6] Depression is strongly associated with increased rates of serious cardiac events, cardiac mortality following myocardial infarction (MI), unstable angina, and coronary artery bypass surgery.[6,28]

Although less well studied than depression, emerging data suggest that anxiety is also an important risk factor for incidence and progression of CVD.[6] Considerable covariation between depression, anxiety, and anger/hostility have been found to increase the risk of CVD through the infliction of a shared general distress.[6] However, anxiety symptoms may increase cardiac risk beyond effects of general distress, suggesting anxiety is a core feature of post-MI depression, and worth considering separately from depression and other psychological risk factors to identify patients at risk for depression following MI.[6] General measures of anxiety and psychological distress have been associated with increased rates of 5-year cardiac-related mortality in patients with MI, with one study showing anxiety more strongly related with subsequent cardiac events than depression or hostility.[6] Chronic anxiety, phobic anxiety, and posttraumatic stress disorder have shown the strongest associations with CVD.[6]

The recent and widely publicized Nurses' Health Study results, however, lend further evidence to the seriousness of depression and its association with fatal cardiac events' outcomes.[28] In this study, women without known cardiovascular disease at baseline and with symptoms of depression had significantly increased risks of 3 coronary heart disease (CHD) events (sudden cardiac death, MI, and fatal CHD), the strongest association seen with fatal CHD, with a relative risk of 1.49 (confidence interval [CI]: 1.11–2.00, P trend = .007).[28] Depressive symptoms were also associated with multiple risk factors for CHD, including history of hypertension, diabetes, high cholesterol, smoking, obesity, being less physically active, and having lower ω-3 fatty acid intake. Clinical depression or use of antidepressant medication showed a 2.33-fold risk of sudden cardiac death (SCD) (CI: 1.47–3.70, $P < .001$), indicating clinically relevant depression is a stronger predictor of SCD than nonclinical depressive symptoms.[28] When examined separately, neither depression score nor antidepressant use was significantly associated with nonfatal cardiac events. The investigators pose an explanation for fatal outcomes as possibly due to an increased risk of ventricular arrhythmias with the use of antidepressant medication. This theory was supported in their data by an elevated risk for SCD in association with antidepressant use, but not with more severe depressive symptoms, and the risk was not reduced when multiple coronary risk factors were adjusted for.

Irritable bowel syndrome (IBS) is one of the most common and well-studied functional gastrointestinal disorders, affects an estimated 10% to 25% of the population, and occurs in women twice as frequently as men.[6] Stress reactivity is considered an important nondiagnostic feature of IBS and is characteristic of other disorders overlapping with IBS, such as anxiety and mood disorders.[6] There is a strong association between IBS and psychiatric diagnoses, with between 54% and 94% of treatment-seeking patients with IBS having a mood or anxiety disorder diagnosis.[6] When psychiatric disorders coexist with IBS, gastrointestinal symptoms are typically more severe and disabling, and those with panic disorder may be up to 5 times more likely to exhibit IBS-like symptoms than those with no psychiatric diagnosis.[6] Up to one-third of IBS patients have posttraumatic stress disorder.[6]

Medical literature shows a strong relationship of IBS with both anxiety and depression, and is sufficiently specific to differentiate a higher frequency of IBS symptoms among those with panic disorder, GAD, and major depressive disorder versus social anxiety disorder, specific phobia, and obsessive-compulsive disorder.[29] Because of the high coincidence between IBS and depression, the role of serotonin in IBS has been widely studied, with antidepressant use in the treatment of IBS more effective than other IBS-specific medications.[29] Cognitive-behavioral therapy has also been instituted with some benefit which, along with antidepressant medicine, supports the "brain-gut disorder" model of disease for IBS.[29]

Obesity in United States adults has increased from about 23% in 1990 to 31% in 2000,[30,31] with two-thirds of the United States adult population either overweight or obese (ie, with a body mass index [BMI], calculated as the weight in kilograms divided by height in meters squared, ≥ 25).[31] Obesity is associated with increases in risk for numerous health outcomes including cardiovascular disease, type 2 diabetes, and some cancers, as well as personal dissatisfaction with one's physical appearance.[31] Obesity also raises the risk of psychopathology among women at clinical and subclinical levels, with the odds of a major depressive episode in the past year increasing by 37% among obese women, with a 22% increase in odds for each 10-unit increase in continuous BMI.[32] Odds for lifetime prevalence of anxiety disorders and mood disorders increases by 34% in obese women when compared with nonobese women.[32]

Long-term impact of obesity on GAD and major depressive disorder (MDD) was found independent of other more substantial risk factors implicated in psychopathology.[32] Obesity has been shown to predict MDD and anxiety, with increasing cumulative stress burden and poor self-concept eventually lowering the threshold at which stress exposure may precipitate depression.[32] A step-wise increase has been seen mutually in BMI and depression, with increasing severity of depressive symptoms having a strong association with higher risk of obesity, and increasing BMI being strongly associated with higher risk of depressive disorder.[30] These associations seem to be consistent across demographic groups and not confounded by age, race, marital status, educational attainment, or tobacco or antidepressant use.[30] Significantly lower activity levels and higher caloric intake also show consistent association with depression.[30]

Vitamin D deficiency has been associated with mood disorders, including MDD and premenstrual syndrome,[33] anxiety disorders,[34] and reduced cognitive function.[34] In an intervention study, overweight and obese subjects tested low in serum 25(OH)D (vitamin D) and higher in depressive scores than those with higher vitamin D levels.[34]

Depressive scores improved after high-dose vitamin D supplementation over a 1-year period of time.[34] The improvement in depressive scores appeared unrelated to age and BMI.

SUMMARY

Depression and anxiety in women across the life span pose a significant burden to the women themselves as well as to the public health system, and costs United States society tens of billions of dollars each year.[8] Depression and anxiety predispose a person to other physical ailments, and physical morbidity can trigger depression or anxiety, often worsening distress. Depression and anxiety may occur in tandem, and during particularly vulnerable periods in a woman's life. Mood and anxiety disorders often present in association with hormonal/endocrine changes such as during puberty, the menstrual cycle, pregnancy, and the menopausal transition. Awareness of issues specific to the presentation of depression and anxiety in women, the comorbidity of psychological and physical disorders, special coping mechanisms women employ in self-management, and awareness of medical assessment and treatment, including complementary and alternative medicine, can result in early detection, education, and intervention, as well as close follow-up to reduce stigma, suffering, and adverse health outcomes in women.

REFERENCES

1. National Institute of Mental Health. Available at: http://www.nimh.nih.gov/health/topics/statistics/index.xhtml. Accessed March 18, 2009.
2. Alexander JL. Quest for timely detection and treatment of women with depression. J Manag Care Pharm 2007;13(9suppl a):S3–11.
3. U.S. Department of Health and Human Services. Mental health: a report of the surgeon general—executive summary. Rockville (MD): U.S. Department of Health and Human Services, Substance Abuse and Mental Health Services Administration, Center for Mental Health Services, National Institutes of Health, National Institute of Mental Health; 1999.
4. Nakamura R. Workshop Report: surgeon general's workshop on women's mental health. Denver, Colorado, 2005.
5. Schreiber R. Understanding and helping depressed women. Arch Psychiatr Nurs 1996;10(3):165–75.
6. Roy-Byrne R, Davidson KW, Kessler RC, et al. Anxiety disorders and comorbid medical illness. Gen Hosp Psychiatry 2008;30:208–25.
7. Peden AR. Up from depression: strategies used by women recovering from depression. J Psychiatr Ment Health Nurs 1994;1:77–83.
8. Meyer BL. A holistic approach to severe depression: my story. Holist Nurs Pract 2008;22(2):81–6.
9. Kim YH, Bowers J. Efficacy of acupuncture for treating depression. Alternative Therapies in Women's Health 2007;9(7):49–56.
10. Klein R. Anxiety disorders. J Child Psychol Psychiatry 2009;50:153–62.
11. Lack CW, Green AL. Mood disorders in children and adolescents. J Pediatr Nurs 2009;24(1):13–25.
12. Victor AM, Bernstein GA. Anxiety disorders and posttraumatic stress disorder update. Psychiatr Clin North Am 2009;32:57–69.
13. Busse JW, Montori VM, Krasnik C, et al. Psychological intervention for premenstrual syndrome: a meta-analysis of randomized controlled trials. Psychother Psychosom 2009;78:6–15.

14. Maki PM. Menopause and anxiety: immediate and long-term effects. Menopause 2008;15(6):1033–5.
15. Stearns S. PMS and PMDD in the domain of mental health nursing. J Psychosoc Nurs Ment Health Serv 2001;30(1):16–27.
16. Yang M, Wallenstein G, Hagan M, et al. Burden of premenstrual dysphoric disorder on health-related quality of life. J Womens Health (Larchmt) 2008; 17(1):113–21.
17. Gold EB, Bair Y, Block G, et al. Diet and lifestyle factors associated with premenstrual symptoms in a racially diverse community sample: study of women's health across the nation (SWAN). J Womens Health (Larchmt) 2007;16(5):641–55.
18. Bowen A, Muhajarine N. Antenatal depression. Cancer Nurs 2006;102(9):27–30.
19. Tezel A, Gozum S. Comparison of effects of nursing care to problem solving training on levels of depressive symptoms in postpartum women. Patient Educ Couns 2006;63:64–73.
20. Mann JR, McKeown RE, Bacon J, et al. Do antenatal religious and spiritual factors impact the risk of postpartum depressive symptoms? J Womens Health (Larchmt) 2008;17(5):745–55.
21. McDowell WK. Health matters: promoting health and wellness. Detecting women at risk for postpartum mood disorders. Nursing 2008;38(3):57–8.
22. Olshansky E, Sereika S. The transition from pregnancy to postpartum in previously infertile women: a focus on depression. Arch Psychiatr Nurs 2005;19(6):273–80.
23. Dunn LL, Handley MC, Shelton MM. Spiritual well-being, anxiety, and depression in antepartal women on bedrest. Issues Ment Health Nurs 2007;28:1235–46.
24. Harsh VL, Rubinow DR, Schmidt PJ. Can the menopausal transition trigger depression? Contemp Ob Gyn 2008;53(8):28–33.
25. Studd J, Panay N. Are oestrogens useful for the treatment of depression in women? Best Pract Res Clin Obstet Gynaecol 2009;23:63–71.
26. Soares CN. Depression during the menopausal transition: window of vulnerability or continuum of risk? Menopause 2008;15(2):207–9.
27. European College of Neuropsychopharmacology. Depression and cardiovascular disease. Science Daily 2007. Available at: http://www.sciencedaily.com/releases/2007/10/071015131515.htm. Accessed April 2, 2009.
28. Whang W, Kubzansky LD, Kawachi I, et al. Depression and risk of sudden cardiac death and coronary heart disease in women. J Am Coll Cardiol 2009; 53:950–8.
29. Curtiss FR. Irritable bowel syndrome and antidepressants. J Manag Care Pharm 2008;14(9):882–5.
30. Simon GE, Ludman EJ, Linde JA, et al. Association between obesity and depression in middle-aged women. Gen Hosp Psychiatry 2008;30:32–9.
31. Annesi JJ, Whitaker AC. Relations of mood and exercise with weight loss in formerly sedentary obese women. Am J Health Behav 2008;32(6):676–83.
32. Kasen S, Cohen P, Chen H, et al. Obesity and psychopathology in women: a three decade prospective study. Int J Obes 2008;32:558–66.
33. Murphy PK, Wagner CL. Vitamin D and mood disorders among women: an integrative review. J Midwifery Womens Health 2008;53(5):440–6.
34. Jorde R, Sneve M, Figenschau Y, et al. Effects of vitamin D supplementation on symptoms of depression in overweight and obese subjects: randomized double blind trial. J Intern Med 2008;264:599–609.

Women Prisoners: Health Issues and Nursing Implications

Anastasia A. Fisher, RN, DNSc[a], Diane C. Hatton, RN, DNSc[b],*

KEYWORDS

• Prisoners • Prisons • Women's health
• Ethnic groups • Female

The purpose of this article is to describe health issues of women prisoners, analyze the implications of these issues for nursing practice, and consider strategies to improve the health of this vulnerable population. The article focuses primarily on women prisoners in the United States and includes a brief contextual background to explain the rapid increase in their numbers. Although the incarceration of women is increasingly a global problem,[1,2] the authors focus primarily on the situation in the United States because discussion of the global incarceration of women is beyond the scope of this article.

BACKGROUND

In 2008, the Pew Center on the States reported that 3 decades of prison growth had led to a new threshold: 1 in every 100 US adults was confined in jail or prison.[3] The Pew report notes that these incarceration rates have left "cash-strapped states with soaring costs they can ill afford" and that incarceration has failed "to have a clear impact on either recidivism or overall crime."[3] US incarceration reflects ethnic and racial disparities; among women, African American women have the highest rates, followed by Hispanic and white women (**Table 1**). In the United States, "A Black woman is more than seven times as likely as a White woman to spend time behind bars."[4] Although more men than women are incarcerated, women's rates have increased more rapidly. For example, in state and federal prisons, the average annual change in the growth rate from 2005 to 2006 was 4.6% for women compared with 2.7% for men; in jails, the number of women has increased at a rate of 4.9% compared with 2.2% for men.[5] Women also comprise 23% of those on probation and 12% of those on parole—approximately 797,000.[6]

[a] School of Nursing, San Francisco State University, 1600 Holloway Avenue, BH 357, San Francisco, CA 94132, USA
[b] School of Nursing, San Diego State University, 5500 Campanile Drive, San Diego, CA 92128, USA
* Corresponding author.
E-mail address: dhatton@mail.sdsu.edu (D.C. Hatton).

Nurs Clin N Am 44 (2009) 365–373
doi:10.1016/j.cnur.2009.06.010
0029-6465/09/$ – see front matter © 2009 Elsevier Inc. All rights reserved.
nursing.theclinics.com

Table 1	
Incarceration rates for US women prisoners aged 35 to 39 years	
Ethnic Group	Incarceration Rate
African American	1 in 100
Hispanic	1 in 297
White	1 in 355

Data from Pew Center on the States, 2008.

Prisons and jails differ from one another in several ways, some of which are important for health. One major difference is that jails typically hold individuals with a sentence of a year or less; but jails also hold those awaiting trial, conviction, or sentencing.[7] Jails witness a more transient population than prisons, and evidence shows that more than 1 million women pass through the nation's jails during a year.[8] Because drug and/or alcohol use is prevalent, withdrawal after arrest is a major concern.[9,10] In most cases, jails are locally operated and have fewer resources than state and federal prisons.

Women serving a sentence of a year or more are usually transferred to a prison. The differences among prisons are further complicated by variations from state to state and from state to federal systems. The largest prison populations are found in the federal prison system followed by the states of Texas, California, Florida, and New York.[11] More detailed discussion of the differences between jails and prisons is beyond the scope of this article; however, the authors use the term "prison" to simplify the discussion, as many of the health problems and their accompanying challenges apply to both types of institutions.

Most woman prisoners are in their thirties and have minor children, few job skills, and limited education. Whereas men in the United States are increasingly incarcerated for violent offenses, this is not usually the case for women, who are often incarcerated for nonviolent drug and property crimes.[12] Often women prisoners come from disadvantaged communities that are medically underserved, they have not seen a health care provider in the past year, and they have limited health care access before arriving in jail or prison.[13] In addition, when compared with men, women who enter jail are more likely to have a history of homelessness, illicit drug use, and multiple health problems.[14]

During the last few decades, US criminal justice policies, especially those related to the War on Drugs and its harsh mandatory sentencing laws, have led to high rates of confinement, rather than community-based alternatives, for women convicted of low-level, nonviolent crimes.[15,16] Discussion about this enormous increase in the number of prisoners frequently focuses on public safety, with little attention to the health needs of prisoners, their families, and their communities. But incarceration severely affects health and well-being; it disproportionately affects women of color, exacerbating their health disparities. Women prisoners "are removed from their communities, they are placed in close proximity to a population of women with high rates of infectious and chronic diseases, and opportunities to link them to needed services are missed."[4]

HEALTH ISSUES AMONG WOMEN PRISONERS

The literature contains excellent accounts of the multiple health problems commonly found among women prisoners.[17] This article, therefore, selects some of the most salient health issues and analyzes their challenges for nursing. The authors consider health from a broad perspective, as does the World Health Organization, focusing on health as a state of "physical, mental, and social well-being."[18] Many of the health concerns discussed later overlap the boundaries of these three categories, but are separated for purposes of this discussion.

Physical Health

Women often arrive at and leave prison with an increased incidence of undertreated chronic physical health problems, including asthma, hypertension, heart disease, and diabetes.[15,19] Histories of substance use or abuse, multiple sexual partners, and inconsistent contraceptive use also place them at high risk for unplanned pregnancies and sexually transmitted diseases (STDs), including human immunodeficiency virus (HIV) and hepatitis B and C.[20] Estimates indicate that 6% to 10% of incarcerated women are pregnant, and approximately 1400 give birth each year.[21] Research also documents that during pregnancy, up to one-half have used alcohol and other drugs.[22,23] In addition, women often report extensive histories of childhood and adult violence, including physical and sexual assault.[24,25] These multiple health risks contribute to complicated pregnancies, childbirth, and mothering.[26]

A full range of gynecologic and obstetric care services for women prisoners is a standard recognized by the American Public Health Association,[27] the National Commission on Correctional Health Care,[28] and the World Health Organization's Health in Prison Project.[29] However, reproductive health of women in prisons is often overlooked.[30] Women report gynecologic examinations performed by providers who are unprofessional and rude and who offer little information in a language they can understand.[31] Research further indicates that abortion services are inconsistent and lack standardization,[32] and that full access to abortion services is not available in all settings.[33] These conditions exist despite legal precedents that establish the right of an incarcerated pregnant woman to decide if she wants to continue her pregnancy.[34]

Innovative programs have demonstrated success in addressing reproductive and other health needs of incarcerated women. Educational support groups led by nurses in prison have improved contraceptive use upon release to the community and reduced unplanned pregnancies.[35] Lamaze educators and doula programs have targeted pregnancy and delivery and demonstrated satisfaction among recipients of care.[36,37] Programs addressing other health concerns include the Well-integrated Screening and Evaluation for Women across the Nation (WISEWOMEN) program in South Dakota that focused on reducing heart disease and stroke risk among women prisoners.[38] In addition to screening and education, this program provides opportunities to link women with services outside prison, upon release.

The health concerns of a growing population of older women prisoners present unique challenges, and evidence suggests that prisons are failing to provide for the health needs of this vulnerable population.[39] The built environment of prisons, including few lower bunks, a lack of handrails in cells, and long distances to dining halls, make it particularly difficult for older women.[40] Reports include accounts of older prisoners falling and being injured during routine prison activities that can include dropping to the ground for alarms and mandatory work in prison programs. Because of these conditions, advocates recommend expanding compassionate release laws to include older prisoners and those with disabilities.[40] Functional assessments, modifications of environmental conditions, and adequate health care are required to meet the needs of older women who remain in prison.[41]

Older prisoners who are terminally ill present a more difficult challenge. Hospice services in prisons have shown success in providing patient comfort and reducing suffering for those who are not granted compassionate release.[42] The Guiding

Responsive Actions for Corrections at End-of-Life (GRACE) project is an example of a program that has as its goal the development of high-quality end-of-life care in prisons and the promotion of a standard of care equal to that of hospice programs in the community.[43]

Mental Health

In addition to their physical health issues, women prisoners also experience a variety of mental health problems. They report high rates of mania, major depression, anxiety (including posttraumatic stress disorder), personality disorders, psychotic disorders, and substance abuse and dependence.[10,44] A recent study by the Bureau of Justice Statistics found that 73% of the women in state prisons and 75% of women in local jails have symptoms of mental disorders, compared with 12% of women in the general population.[45] Three-quarters of the women with a mental health problem also met criteria for substance abuse or dependence. Comorbidity of substance-use disorders and other psychiatric problems is common among women prisoners.[10] Comorbidity is associated with increased risk for STDs, HIV/AIDS, homelessness, and more rapid return to incarceration once released to the community.[44,46]

Although jails and prisons were never intended to be mental hospitals, they have become the nation's largest psychiatric facilities.[47,48] There are now more individuals with severe mental illness in the Los Angeles County Jail, Chicago's Cook County Jail, or New York's Rikers Island Jail than there are in any single psychiatric hospital in the nation.[49] Because jails and prisons are ill equipped to deal with persons who have mental health problems, they often fail to provide adequate services to those experiencing complex, multiple disorders. Prison mental health is focused on managing crisis and symptoms rather than providing treatment for psychiatric problems.[50] Inadequate mental health and substance abuse treatment services and the harsh conditions of incarceration contribute to adverse consequences for women prisoners. These include longer sentences and prolonged isolation, hopelessness, self-mutilation, violence, and suicide.[50]

As long as persons with mental health and substance abuse problems are incarcerated, treatment services within US jails and prisons must be improved; however, the cost of providing adequate services to this growing population of prisoners is significant. One alternative to the continued incarceration of nonviolent women prisoners with serious psychiatric problems is the mental health court. Mental health courts divert individuals with mental health problems from jail or standard probation to supervised treatment programs for a fixed length of time. Currently, there are about 175 mental health courts in the United States.[51] This alternative requires further investment in the community mental health system, one that addresses issues of poverty and homelessness among women prisoners and one where access to mental health and substance abuse treatment is readily available on demand.[50]

Social Health

Since 1991, the number of women in state and federal prisons who have minor children increased 131%. Before incarceration, more than half of the mothers were the family's primary financial support. Among the women who lived with their minor children before imprisonment (64%), 9% reported homelessness the year before incarceration, 73% reported a mental health problem, and 64% reported substance dependence or abuse. When a mother goes to prison, the care for her children is transferred to grandparents (44.9%), the other parent (37%), other relatives (22.8%), a foster home (10.9%), or others (7.8%).[52]

Maintaining contact with minor children and other family members is often difficult for women prisoners. One factor contributing to this situation is the geographic isolation of many women's prisons. Because there are smaller numbers of women in prison than men, states have fewer facilities to house women. For example, in California, the Central California Women's Facility (CCWF)[53] and the Valley State Prison for Women (VSPW)[54] are located adjacent to each other in the central part of the state at some distance from major metropolitan areas. These prisons, which (as of this writing) house 7903 women, were originally designed for 4028. Periodically, children are able to access free travel to these prisons to visit their mothers through the "Get on the Bus" program, which provides transportation and meals for the day. If they live in San Francisco, the 152-mile trip takes approximately 2.5 hours; from San Diego, the 377-mile trip takes nearly 6 hours. This case illustrates how remote women's prisons can be from families and community resources. Not surprisingly, almost one-third of women in the nation's state and federal prisons report that they have contact with their children only monthly or even less often.[52]

Some states have implemented prisoner/mother programs, whereby mothers are allowed to transfer to a facility where they can have custody of children. However, critics note that these programs can serve as vehicles for social control rather than helping mothers parent their children.[55] If mothers are able to complete their prison term without losing custody of their children, they may still find it difficult to keep their family relationships intact in states that prohibit those convicted of a felony to obtain services such as food stamps, public housing, and loans for school.[56] These are only a few of the many challenges women face upon release; yet research demonstrates that children often remain a central focus for women. Richie[57] argues that with adequate support, even a noncustodial relationship with a child is an important stabilizing force for women as they transition to the community.

In summary, research evidence documents how mass incarceration contributes to poor physical, mental, and social health among women prisoners; also documented is the difficulty women encounter accessing health care in prison.[4,58–62] They experience a myriad of health problems while incarcerated, and they return to their communities with untreated, serious health problems that place a substantial burden on the already financially stressed health care systems.[19] This situation is further compounded by soaring prison health care costs. In 2008, the State of California spent more than $2.1 billion on health care in prisons—a 210% increase since 2000.[3] Despite expenditures, in 2005, US District Court Judge Thelton Henderson found that the California health care system was "broken beyond repair…the threat of future injury and death is virtually guaranteed in the absence of drastic action."[63] The judge then placed the health care in California's prison system under the jurisdiction of a Federal Receiver. In contrast to the situation in the United States, the movement in the United Kingdom has been to integrate prison health care into the National Health Service. The intent is that the standard of care provided to prisoners should be the same as that provided to the general population.[64]

IMPROVING THE HEALTH OF WOMEN PRISONERS

Delivering safe nursing care to women prisoners requires gender-sensitive strategies[12] and consideration of their extraordinary vulnerability.[65] Nurse authors have addressed the roles, the complexity, and the many dilemmas faced when working with prisoners.[15,66–69] Clearly, good prison health is good public health,[70] and nurses working in prisons have a vital role to play in promoting health among members of this vulnerable population.

Although the authors clearly recognize that nursing practice within prisons and jails is highly complex, rather than focusing on this complexity, they choose to take a more upstream approach that involves moving beyond the current system and developing strong partnerships with others. Building on the work of Freudenberg,[4] the authors recommend that nurses develop partnerships with jails/prisons to assure that adequate health and social services are provided in their facilities. They also recommend strengthening reentry programs for women that include health care, housing, parenting, education, and employment. Finally, they recommend, as does Richie,[57] upstream strategies for addressing the issues of incarceration of women that target the disadvantaged communities from which many women prisoners come:

> The challenges women face must be met with expanded opportunity and a more thoughtful criminal justice policy. This would require a plan for reinvestment in low-income communities in this country that centers on women's needs for safety and self-sufficiency. If undertaken, such a reform agenda might even prevent some of the arrests and incarcerations of women from low-income communities in the first place.[57]

REFERENCES

1. Walmsley R. World female imprisonment list. International Centre for Prison Studies. Available at: http://www.unodc.org/pdf/india/womens_corner/women_prison_list_2006.pdf. Accessed May 16, 2009.
2. Sudbury J, editor. Global lockdown. Race, gender, and the prison-industrial complex. New York: Routledge; 2005.
3. The Pew Center on the States. One in 100: behind bars in America 2008. Pew Charitable Trusts. Available at: http://www.pewcenteronthestates.org/uploadedFiles/One%20in%20100.pdf. Accessed May 14, 2009.
4. Freudenberg N. Adverse effects of US jail and prison policies on the health and well-being of women of color. Am J Public Health 2002;92(12):1895–9.
5. Sabol WJ, Minton TD, Harrison PM. Prison and jail inmates at midyear 2006. Bureau of Justice Statistics. Available at: http://www.ojp.usdoj.gov/bjs/pub/pdf/pjim06.pdf. Accessed May 15, 2009.
6. Glaze LE, Bonczar TP. Probation and parole in the United States, 2007 statistical tables. Bureau of Justice Statistics. Available at: http://www.ojp.gov/bjs/pub/pdf/ppus07st.pdf. Accessed May 14, 2009.
7. Harrison PM, Beck AJ. Prison and jail inmates at midyear 2005. Bureau of Justice Statistics. Available at: http://www.ojp.usdoj.gov/bjs/pub/pdf/pjim05.pdf. Accessed March 1, 2008.
8. Richie BE, Freudenberg N, Page J. Reintegrating women leaving jail into urban communities: a description of a model program. J Urban Health 2001;78(2):290–303.
9. Kane M, DiBartolo M. Complex physical and mental health needs of rural incarcerated women. Issues Ment Health Nurs 2002;23(3):209–29.
10. Abram KM, Teplin LA, McClelland GM. Comorbidity of severe psychiatric disorders and substance use disorders among women in jail. Am J Psychiatry 2003; 160(5):1007–10.
11. West HC, Sabol W. Prison inmates at midyear 2008–statistical tables. Bureau of Justice Statistics. Available at: http://www.ojp.gov/bjs/pub/pdf/pim08st.pdf. Accessed May 14, 2009.
12. Bloom B, Owen B, Covington S, et al. Gender-responsive strategies. Research, practice, and guiding principles for women offenders, vol. 2008. Washington, DC: National Institute of Corrections; 2003.

13. Conklin TJ, Lincoln T, Tuthill RW. Self-reported health and prior health behaviors of newly admitted correctional inmates. Am J Public Health 2000;90(12):1939–41.
14. Freudenberg N, Moseley J, Labriola M, et al. Comparison of health and social characteristics of people leaving New York city jails by age, gender, and race/ethnicity: implications for public health interventions. Public Health Rep 2007; 122(6):733–43.
15. Maeve MK. Nursing care partnerships with women leaving jail. Effects on health and crime. J Psychosoc Nurs Ment Health Serv 2003;41(9):30–40.
16. Walmsley R. Prison planet. Foreign Pol 2007;160:30–1.
17. Braithwaite RL, Arriola KJ, Newkirk C. Health issues among incarcerated women. New Jersey: Rutgers University Press; 2006.
18. World Health Organization. WHO definition of health. Available at: http://www.who.int/about/definition/en/print.html. Accessed May 14, 2009.
19. National Commission on Correctional Health Care. The health status of soon-to-be-released inmates. A report to Congress. National Commission on Correctional Health Care. Available at: http://www.ncchc.org/pubs/pubs_stbr.html. Accessed May 17, 2009.
20. Clarke JG, Hebert MR, Rosengard C, et al. Reproductive health care and family planning needs among incarcerated women. Am J Public Health 2006;96(5): 834–9.
21. Clarke JG, Rosengard C, Rose J, et al. Pregnancy attitudes and contraceptive plans among women entering jail. Women Health 2006;43(2):111–30.
22. Fogel CI, Belyea M. The lives of incarcerated women: violence, substance abuse, and at risk for HIV. J Assoc Nurses AIDS Care 1999;10(6):66–74.
23. Fogel CI, Belyea M. Psychological risk factors in pregnant inmates. A challenge for nursing. MCN Am J Matern Child Nurs 2001;26(1):10–6.
24. Browne A, Miller B, Maguin E. Prevalence and severity of lifetime physical and sexual victimization among incarcerated women. Int J Law Psychiatry 1999; 22(3–4):301–22.
25. Fickenscher A, Lapidus J, Silk-Walker P, et al. Women behind bars: health needs of inmates in a county jail. Public Health Rep 2001;116:191–6.
26. Peternelj-Taylor C. Pregnancy, childbirth, and mothering: a forensic nursing response. J Forensic Nurs 2008;4(2):53–4.
27. American Public Health Association Task Force on Correctional Health Care Standards. Standards for health services in correctional institutions. Washington, DC: American Public Health Association; 2003.
28. National Commission on Correctional Health Care. Position statements: women's health care in correctional settings. Available at: http://www.ncchc.org/resources/statements/womenshealth2005.html. Accessed May 14, 2009.
29. World Health Organization. Women's health in prison. Available at: http://www.euro.who.int/Document/E92347.pdf. Accessed May 16, 2009.
30. Braithwaite RL, Treadwell HM, Arriola KR. Health disparities and incarcerated women: a population ignored. Am J Public Health 2005;95(10):1679–81.
31. Magee CG, Hult JR, Turalba R, et al. Preventive care for women in prison: a qualitative community health assessment of the Papanicolaou test and follow-up treatment at a California state women's prison. Am J Public Health 2005;95(10): 1712–7.
32. Roth R. Do prisoners have abortion rights? Fem Stud 2004;30(2):353–81.
33. Sufrin CB, Creinin MD, Chang JC. Incarcerated women and abortion provision: a survey of correctional health providers. Perspect Sex Reprod Health 2009; 41(1):6–11.

34. Kasdan D. Abortion access for incarcerated women: are correctional health practices in conflict with constitutional standards? Perspect Sex Reprod Health 2009; 41(1):59–62.

35. Ferszt GG, Erickson-Owens DA. Development of an educational/support group for pregnant women in prison. J Forensic Nurs 2008;4(2):55–60.

36. Hotelling BA. Perinatal needs of pregnant, incarcerated women. J Perinat Educ 2008;17(2):37–44.

37. Schroeder C, Bell J. Doula birth support for incarcerated pregnant women. Public Health Nurs 2005;22(1):53–8.

38. Khavjou OA, Clarke J, Hofeldt RM, et al. A captive audience: bringing the WISE-WOMAN program to South Dakota prisoners. Womens Health Issues 2007;17(4): 193–201.

39. Reviere R, Young VD. Aging behind bars: health care for older female inmates. J Women Aging 2004;16(1/2):55–69.

40. Strupp H, Willmott D. Dignity denied: the price of imprisoning older women in California legal services for prisoners with children. Available at: http://www. prisonerswithchildren.org/pubs/dignity.pdf. Accessed May 14, 2009.

41. Williams BA, Lindquist K, Sudore RL, et al. Being old and doing time: functional impairment and adverse experiences of geriatric female prisoners. J Am Geriatr Soc 2006;54(4):702–7.

42. Linder JF, Enders SR, Craig E, et al. Hospice care for the incarcerated in the United States: an introduction. J Palliat Med 2002;5(4):549–52.

43. Volunteers of America. Guiding responsive action for corrections at end-of-life (GRACE). Available at: http://www.mywhatever.com/cifwriter/library/41/pe1260. html. Accessed May 14, 2009.

44. Covington S. Women and the criminal justice system. Womens Health Issues 2007;17:180–2.

45. James DJ, Glaze LE. Mental health problems of prison and jail inmates. US Department of Justice. Available at: http://ojp.usdoj.gov/bjs/pub/pdf/mhppji. pdf. Accessed March 1, 2008.

46. Fearn NE, Parker K. Health care for women inmates: issues, perceptions and policy considerations. Californian J Health Promot 2005;3(2):1–22.

47. Hatton DC, Fisher AA. Incarceration and the new asylums: consequences for the mental health of women prisoners. Issues Ment Health Nurs 2008;29(12):1304–7.

48. Public Broadcasting System (PBS). The new asylums. WGBH Educational Foundation; 2005.

49. Treatment Advocacy Center. Criminalization of individuals with severe psychiatric disorders. Available at: http://www.treatmentadvocacycenter.org/. Accessed May 15, 2009.

50. Human Rights Watch. Ill-equipped: prisons and offenders with mental illness. Available at: http://www.hrw.org/reports/2003/usa1003/index.htm. Accessed May 15, 2009.

51. Schwartz E. How special courts can serve justice and help mentally ill offenders. Available at: http://www.usnews.com/articles/news/national/2008/02/07/mental-health-courts.html. Accessed May 15, 2009.

52. Glaze LE, Maruschak LM. Parents in prison and their minor children. Available at: http://www.ojp.usdoj.gov/bjs/pub/pdf/pptmc.pdf. Accessed May 14, 2009.

53. California Department of Corrections and Rehabilitation. Central California Women's Facility (CCWF). Available at: http://www.cdcr.ca.gov/Visitors/Facilities/CCWF.html. Accessed May 14, 2009.

54. California Department of Corrections and Rehabilitation. Valley State Prison for Women (VSPW). Available at: http://www.cdcr.ca.gov/Visitors/Facilities/VSPW. html. Accessed May 14, 2009.

55. Craig SC. A historical review of mother and child programs for incarcerated women. Prison J 2009;89:35S–53S.
56. Roth R. Prisons as sites of reproductive injustice. Off Our Backs 2006;36(4): 69–71.
57. Richie B. Challenges incarcerated women face as they return to their communities: findings from life history interviews. Crime Delinq 2001;47(3):368–89.
58. Hatton DC, Kleffel D, Fisher AA. Prisoners' perspectives of health problems and healthcare in a US women's jail. Women Health 2006;44(1):119–36.
59. Willmott D, van Olphen J. Challenging the health impacts of incarceration: the role for community health workers. Californian J Health Promot 2005;3(2):38–48.
60. Stoller N. Improving access to health care for California's women prisoners. University of California/The California Policy Research Center. Available at: http://www.ucop.edu/cprc/stollerpaper.pdf. Accessed May 25, 2005.
61. Stoller N. Space, place and movement as aspects of health care in three women's prisons. Soc Sci Med 2003;56(11):2263–75.
62. Massoglia M. Incarceration as exposure: the prison, infectious disease, and other stress-related illnesses. J Health Soc Behav 2008;49(1):56–71.
63. California Prison Healthcare Receivership Corp. About us. California Prison Healthcare Services. Available at: http://www.cphcs.ca.gov/about.aspx. Accessed August 17, 2008.
64. Watson R. Editoral: prison healthcare. J Clin Nurs 2007;16:1195.
65. Peternelj-Taylor C. Incarceration of vulnerable populations. J Psychosoc Nurs Ment Health Serv 2003;41(9):4–5.
66. Peternelj-Taylor C. Forensic psychiatric nursing: the paradox of custody and caring. J Psychosoc Nurs Ment Health Serv 1999;37(9):9–11.
67. Norman AE, Parrish AA. Prison nursing. Oxford (UK): Blackwell; 2002.
68. Maeve MK, Vaughn MS. Nursing with prisoners: the practice of caring, forensic nursing or penal harm nursing? Adv Nurs Sci 2001;24(2):47–64.
69. Droes NS. Correctional nursing practice. J Community Health Nurs 1994;11(4): 201–10.
70. Gatherer A, Moller L, Hayton P. The World Health Organization European Health in Prisons Project after 10 years: persistent barriers and achievements. Am J Public Health 2005;95(10):1696–700.

Global Women's Health: A Spotlight on Caregiving

Judith A. Berg, PhD, RN, WHNP-BC, FAAN, FAANP[a],*,
Nancy Fugate Woods, PhD, RN, FAAN[b]

KEYWORDS

- Women's global health • Informal caregiving
- Millennium development goals
- Economic and health consequences of caregiving
- Gender roles

In the last few decades gender disparities in health and mortality have been recognized in both industrialized nations and those with developing economies. The most commonly cited factors underlying health disparities are poverty, lack of educational opportunities, low social and socioeconomic status, racism, sexism, heterosexism, environmental hazards, and sociocultural or political stressors related to marginalization and health risk behaviors such as tobacco, alcohol, and substance abuse.[1,2] Health disparities and their causes vary both between and within nations and are not solely determined by biological factors and reproduction but also by work load, nutrition, stress, war, and migration, as well as other factors.[3] The purpose of this article is to discuss women's health issues globally and their clinical implications. To illustrate health issues related to workload and stress, a focus on caregiving and resultant consequences is provided.

GLOBAL WOMEN'S HEALTH

The United Nations General Assembly's Millennium Development Goals (MDGs) included internationally agreed-upon targets to improve the health and quality of life for all.[4] Specifically, the eight goals were to (1) eradicate extreme poverty and hunger; (2) achieve universal primary education; (3) promote gender equality and empower women; (4) reduce child mortality; (5) improve maternal health; (6) combat human immunodeficiency virus (HIV)/AIDS, malaria, and other diseases; (7) ensure environmental sustainability; and (8) develop a global partnership for development. In a recent report from the United Nations, some midpoint key successes were highlighted. For

---

[a] University of Arizona College of Nursing, 37565 S. Stoney Cliff Court, Tucson, AZ 85739, USA
[b] University of Washington School of Nursing, Box 357262, Seattle, WA 98195, USA
* Corresponding author.
E-mail address: jberg@nursing.arizona.edu (J.A. Berg).

Nurs Clin N Am 44 (2009) 375–384
doi:10.1016/j.cnur.2009.06.003
0029-6465/09/$ – see front matter © 2009 Elsevier Inc. All rights reserved.

example, absolute poverty is predicted to be reduced by half worldwide and primary school enrollment is at least 90% in all but two regions. The gender parity index in primary education is 95% or higher in 6 of the 10 regions. Improvements have been made to achievement of MDG number 6 through reduction in deaths from measles and AIDS, with the number of newly infected people with HIV declining from 3 million in 2001 to 2.7 million in 2007. Malaria prevention is expanding and incidence of tuberculosis is expected to be halted by 2015. Progress has been made toward reducing global climate change, and economic improvements have allowed developing nations to allocate more resources to poverty reduction. With private sector support, some critical pharmaceuticals and mobile phone technology have spread throughout the developing world.[4] Together these successes have been achieved through expanded efforts via targeted interventions and programs. However, greater effort is required for achievement of MDGs by the target date of 2015, particularly those goals that disproportionately affect women.

Only two of the MDGs specifically relate to women and only one focuses on or specifies women's health. Nevertheless, all eight goals clearly intersect with the health and lives of women.[5] All eight MDGs interweave, and their achievement is interdependent. For example, women are disproportionately represented among the world's poor, and eradication of poverty and hunger, as well as empowerment of women, is critical to advancing women's health. One cannot be successfully achieved without the other. The target of gender equality and empowerment of women requires education, a key to achievement. Reducing child mortality has implications for female children, particularly in cultures with strong male child preference. Improving maternal health by reducing maternal morbidity and mortality has obvious implications for improving women's health overall. Combating HIV/AIDS and other infectious diseases is necessary to improve women's health, not only because these diseases affect women but because women are more commonly the informal caregivers of infected individuals and experience unequal burden from this role, for example, caring for AIDS orphans after having cared for their dying parents. In addition, morbidities specific to women such as breast and cervical cancer, although not mentioned in the MDGs, are essential goals for improving health and achieving gender equality. Environmental sustainability has potential for positively affecting the health of women by ensuring access to food and clean water. Achieving a global partnership for development is essential to promoting access to economic and health care resources and to providing a legal framework that promotes gender equality and protects the rights of the poor and disenfranchised.[5]

Most of the MDGs were hypothesized to have a profoundly positive impact on girls and women, but due to the current global economic slowdown, global climate change, and food crisis, disproportionate effects on the poor are predicted. Because women are disproportionately impoverished, it is unlikely that gender equality will be achieved by 2015.[4,5] Further, disproportionate expectations related to caregiving continue to have a negative effect on women's health and potential for economic parity with their male counterparts worldwide.

CAREGIVING: A GLOBAL WOMEN'S HEALTH ISSUE

The term *informal caregiver* refers to those who provide care or assistance without pay to people who are ill or need help with personal activities of daily living.[6] Caregiving is often a women's health issue, because more women than men are informal caregivers in virtually every nation. In the United States, three out of four caregivers are women, many of whom care simultaneously for aging parents, family members, and children or adolescents.[7] Studies of caregiver characteristics in the home setting illustrate that women, mostly daughters, wives, and mothers, provide the majority of informal care in the community.[8] In Australia, 56% of carers are female, and of this group 38% are in the 35- to 54-year-old age range, whose caring responsibilities may include one or more parents, a partner, and children.[9] In Taiwan, the culture mandates families to care for their family members when disabled or sick[10] and in a study of care of persons with stroke or Alzheimer disease, 66% (n = 68) of caregivers were women.[11] At present, almost two-thirds of employed women in the developing world are in vulnerable jobs as own-account or unpaid family workers.[4]

Caregiving related to gender role socialization, burden, and health consequences has been discussed in the literature. Together this body of work paints a picture demonstrating some positive but mainly negative consequences to the health of women as a result of their caregiving obligations.

GENDER ROLE SOCIALIZATION AND CAREGIVING

Studies of family caregiving document that the bulk of care is provided by women: wives to husbands, daughters to mothers and fathers, sisters to both sisters and brothers. Women are ordered to care by social convention. Gender role socialization creates expectations that the women in families will assume responsibility for elder as well as child caregiving. Indeed, much of society is structured around the constructed arrangements of division of labor in families in which a woman is constantly available to provide volunteer hours that support many social agencies like schools, nursing homes, and so forth. As a result of the assumption that women are available to do this work voluntarily and without pay, much of the work of caregiving remains hidden and has not been accounted for in estimating the cost of home care and other services that rely on women's unpaid work. In addition, women who do not participate in caregiving or other voluntary activities are made to feel guilty about their unwillingness to do so, whereas men are assigned neither responsibility nor accountability for this work.

Because women's workplace participation has been shaped by gender role attitudes, that is, beliefs about what is appropriate for women to do, women have been overrepresented in the lower paying, lower status occupations. For example, in the United States following World War II, women were encouraged to stay at home and if they were employed, the assumption was that their incomes were discretionary and in addition to a man's income to support the family. Even within the professions, such as medicine, women are overrepresented in lower paying strata such as family medicine, and underrepresented in fields such as transplant surgery or neurosurgery. When families must make decisions about who can most readily assume caregiving responsibility for another family member, it is often the woman's income, which is typically lower than her husband's, that is seen as most expendable.

Often the consequences of this social arrangement include lost opportunity costs for women who may need to reduce their employment commitments or leave their paid work to provide care for their families. Linked to loss of employment is loss of accrual of social security benefits for women's own retirement and employee benefits packages that may include retirement benefits and health insurance coverage. Absence from the workplace often places women in jeopardy when they attempt to reenter the workforce even after short absences. In a technologically advanced workplace, women who are not continuously employed face the challenge of reentering jobs that have changed rapidly even during short-term absences. Thus they miss opportunities for training and advancement and their performance level may be compromised because of these lost opportunities. In addition, the loss of opportunities linked to participation in an occupational and social network may limit women's chances at future occupational advancement. As a result, women suffer financially, professionally or occupationally, and socially.

In many Western countries, workplaces have not made adequate adjustments to the dramatic change in workplace participation that now characterizes most contemporary women's lives. Most American women now remain in their occupations during the years in which they are bearing and raising children. In the United States, despite the fact that more than 39% of preschool children's mothers are employed, the increase in work-place-based child care has not kept pace with women's needs.[12] Family leave policies for child care have not matched the generous paid leave assured to support families in many of the Scandinavian countries.[13] Moreover, women's responsibility for eldercare has been recognized only recently, and consequently attention to the consequences of caring for elders for the well-being of the caregiver is limited.

CAREGIVING BURDEN

In Canada, a consequence of reform to the Canadian health care system is a shift in caregiving responsibilities from institutions to communities, in particular to families.[14] The primary effect of this shift is on women, who provide 80% of care to spouses and parents. In addition, 19% of women aged 45 to 64 years in Canada are caregivers.[15] The shift to family care is reported to be a consequence of assumptions that female family members willingly provide the labor and love of caring and that the quality of care by the family is superior.[14] Often unacknowledged is that health care cost cutting, including shorter hospital stays, has a negative impact on women as a result of increased workload added to the myriad of existing responsibilities, including full- or part-time employment, managing households, childrearing, and so forth. For rural women caregivers in Canada, the unique challenges and multiple roles they occupy simultaneously can lead to burnout.[16] Reforms in health care aimed at cost cutting have led to early hospital discharge for many patients, including those who have sustained critical illness or injury.[8] In Korea, institutional provision of care services and facilities for older people is limited, with consequent heavy reliance on family caregivers,[17] and in a study of correlates of caregiver burden, 62.4% (n = 302) of caregivers were women.[18]

The relationship between labor force participation and informal caregiving by women is not completely clear. Berecki-Gisolf and colleagues reported findings from the Australian Longitudinal Study on Women's Health from 2001 (n = 11,202) and 2004 (n = 10,906), and among women taking up care (≥ 7 h/wk) between 2001 and 2004, the number of hours spent in paid employment in 2001 was negatively correlated with hours spent caring in 2004.[19] The study demonstrated that reduced workforce participation was more common for women taking up caregiving than for other women; caregiving may accelerate women's departure from the workforce. The effect of moving from paid employment to unpaid, the key characteristic of informal caregiving, has not been thoroughly investigated. However, one can hypothesize there are economic and social effects related to this shift. Alternatively, women with full- or part-time paid employment may be less available for informal caregiving, or caregiving may be an additional burden or responsibility. Either scenario implies caregiving adds economic or workload burden, and very often both. Hochschild labeled women's work at home as the "second shift," having discovered gender disparity in the amount of work at home in families with 2 employed adults.[20] In addition, studies of work-related stress revealed that whereas men's norepinephrine levels declined when they returned home from work, women's rose.[21]

Caregiving burden on women is not limited to industrialized nations. In Africa, especially sub-Saharan African countries with a high rate of HIV and AIDS, caregiving has increased the workload and economic marginality of women.[22] In Tanzania, caregivers experience physical hardships related to patient personal care and hygiene, fetching water from outside the home, and economic hardships related to relocation and lack of paid employment.[22] In this context, women's burden of work was drastically increased by informal caregiving as was their marginality based on stigma and economic hardships.

Although caregiving is burdensome, it is also a source of meaning and purpose in life for some. Some family members report improved well-being linked to personal growth and satisfaction from caregiving.[23–25] It is important for clinicians and researchers to look beyond burden to assess what fosters women to find gratification in caregiving. It is likely that access to support, respite, and other resources that minimize the stress of caregiving will be important.

HEALTH CONSEQUENCES OF CAREGIVING

There is an extensive body of literature that examines the health of caregivers,[6] and caregiving has been identified as a chronic stressor that places caregivers at risk of health problems.[26,27] Negative health consequences have been attributed to a stress reaction manifested in deteriorating physical and mental health, especially when resources for caregiving are not sufficient.[25] For example, social change, traditional expectations for caregiving, and scarce public resources can cause conflict between modern Japanese women's traditional roles and their current opportunities and values.[28,29] These conflicts are additional stressors, especially when superimposed on multiple role expectations.

In many cases, caregivers are older and have preexisting health problems that may be exacerbated by caregiving activities.[30] Moreover, informal caregiving is known to restrict personal life, social life, and employment of the caregiver, and these factors add additional strain.[31] Early studies demonstrated caregivers have less time to spend with friends, to fulfill other family obligations, or to pursue leisure time activities.[32,33] In addition, caregivers may neglect their own health to provide care for their ill relatives and believe they are not entitled to personal time.[34]

Caregivers have poorer physical and psychological health than people who do not provide care,[31,35] and psychological and physical health appear to be significantly related.[36] Previous investigations of the disparities in health outcomes of caregiving have examined the effects of social support and access to services, with inconsistent results.[23,24] Studies of the effects of discharge from the intensive care unit to general hospital care indicate that both patients and families experience apprehension, anxiety, depression, and confusion.[37] Considering this transfer anxiety, it is possible that discharge from general hospital care to home care by a family member has potential for similar problems. It has been reported that increased caregiver strain is directly related to increased time needed to care for a person with a neurologic disorder[38] and to the stress of caregiving for patients post cardiac surgery.[39,40] Female informal caregivers for people with HIV/AIDS in the Democratic Republic of Congo are primarily women reported to have poor health because of low income, rented accommodation, and little support.[41]

Psychological Health

Hundreds of studies have assessed the effects of caregiving on psychological health.[42] A substantial number demonstrate that caregiving to an older family member is associated with increased psychological distress.[31] Most studies report increased anxiety, depression, and other forms of psychological morbidity related to both the duration and intensity of the caregiving role.[43–45] In contrast, other studies suggest psychological morbidity in caregivers is more closely related to psychological distress from the significant mental health problems of the person being cared for.[46,47] Younger caregivers and spouses report more caregiver burden and depression, but older caregivers, with a higher percentage of women, reported even higher levels of depression with lower levels of self-efficacy.[31] In a meta-analysis by Pinquart and Sorensen, the strongest negative effects of caregiving were observed for clinician-rated depression.[31]

Overall, there is strong evidence that caregivers report more psychological morbidity than noncaregivers, and this may be due to workload, economic conditions, relationship to the person being cared for,[14] multiple role expectations, and a variety of other factors. In developing nations, caregiving tasks may cause more strain due to economic conditions, sanitation difficulties, and lack of access to medication, health care, or goods and services necessary to provide daily living tasks. Poverty, marginalization, and stigma attached to disease and illness can also play an important role.

Physical Health

According to narrative reviews, between 18% and 35% of informal caregivers perceive their health to be fair to poor.[48] Informal caregivers have poorer physical health than noncaregivers as measured by perceived health and by objective health measures such as stress hormones, antibodies, and medication use.[31,49] It is hypothesized that psychological distress, including caregiver burden and depression, may cause negative hormonal changes, increase susceptibility to infectious agents, and cause negative changes to daily living patterns, such as getting insufficient sleep or not maintaining healthy eating.[49,50] In addition, depressed caregivers are known to overreport physical problems.[51] In one qualitative study of the health of caregivers of children with disabilities, the caregivers attributed their poor health to the time, family, and self-care costs of caregiving.[52]

The relationship of caregiving to mortality is not clear. Schulz and Beach found that older spousal caregivers living with a spouse and exhibiting mental and emotional strain had a 63% greater risk of mortality within 4 years than noncaregiving subjects.[53] Yet a large population study (n = 1,137,334) in Northern Ireland found that 4 years following the census, 1.9% of caregivers died compared with 3.5% of the cohort as a whole.[6] However, the relationship between caregiving and mortality was not modified by age or initial health status; therefore, the effects of caregiving could differ for individuals more vulnerable because of advanced age or previous poor health.

Although the link between caregiving and physical health of the caregiver is less clear, it is notable that caregivers frequently report their overall health as only fair to poor. It is not known how the type of caregiving (eg, for elders, those with dementia, or children with disabilities) affects women's physical health. In particular, older caregivers may approach caregiving activities with poor health status or disabilities, which increase the caregiving burden. On the other hand, the meaning of caregiving may provide some women with a reason to live, and may account for their mortality advantage.[23]

CLINICAL IMPLICATIONS OF CAREGIVING

Most informal caregivers are women and primarily family members, and their tasks require time and energy over long periods.[54] Caregiving often involves activities that are physically, emotionally, socially, or financially challenging.[54] The demands of the caregiving role frequently outweigh resources, which results in stress.[55] Because caregiving has potentially deleterious effects on psychological and physical health, it is essential to assess these in current caregivers. Nurses who interface with care-givers and clinicians who provide care either to the caregiver or to the individual she cares for must obtain a thorough history that includes caregiving burden, social support networks, and emotional and physical issues related to caring. Barriers to well-being of the caregiver must be carefully assessed. The result of these assess-ments must lead to specific suggestions for remedies, such as therapeutic interven-tions for mood disorders, community resources that provide information and caregiver support services, suggestions for activities known to promote health in care-givers (such as increased physical activity and healthy eating), and creative strategies that promote use of support networks, such as family and friends. Although these remedies have been examined in the literature,[14,52,56,57] little attention has been given to those caregivers who find meaning and purpose in their informal caregiving. Studies of correlates of well-being in these individuals may uncover key ingredients that can be used to bolster the health and well-being of caregivers who experience more negative health consequences of the caregiving role.

ECONOMIC IMPLICATIONS

What would happen if the federal bailout in the United States were to extend to compensate family caregivers for work that does not now count in the gross domestic product? The current system of volunteer family caregiving lets insurance companies off the hook for providing funding for services delivered by non–family members. Lost opportunity costs for women have not been factored into the real cost of caregiving. It is possible that women find themselves in a cycle in which they provide caregiving for a family member, lose opportunities for income and retirement and health insurance benefits, cycle down into poverty, develop the need for care, and then become recip-ients of caregiving that cannot be provided by their family members, funded by government sources. The calculus of women's original contributions ignores their true economic value.

SUMMARY

Overall achievement of the MDGs has important considerations for informal caregivers globally. It is possible that by acquiring sufficient education, eradicating poverty, promoting gender equality and empowering women, improving maternal health, decreasing communicable diseases, ensuring environmental sustainability, and developing global partnerships, women caregivers could enjoy access to resources that reduce caregiver burden and promote health and well-being. Without the achieve-ment of these goals or recognition of the social and economic burden assumed by women as informal caregivers, gender equality and economic parity cannot be real-ized. Until economic and social parity are achieved, women around the world will continue to experience undue burden, lost opportunities, and health care systems that take advantage of their volunteer caregiving, which likely creates overall negative health consequences.

REFERENCES

1. Burke A, Sheilds W. Millennium development goals: slow movement threatens women's health in developing countries. Editorial. Contraception 2005;72:247–9.

2. Woods NF. A global imperative: development, safety, and health from girl child to woman. International Council on Women's Health Issues semi-annual conference. Gabarone, Botswana, July 9–11, 2008.

3. Van der Kwaak A. Women and health. Vena J 1991;3(1):2–33.

4. U.N. Millenium Development Goals Report (UN MDG Report). United Nations. Available at: http://www.un.org/milleniumdevelopmentgoalsreport2008/. Accessed March 22, 2009.

5. Shaw D. Women's right to health and the Millennium Development Goals: promoting partnerships to improve access. Int J Gynaecol Obstet 2006;94: 207–15.

6. O'Reilly D, Connolly S, Rosato M, et al. Is caring associated with an increased risk of mortality? A longitudinal study. Soc Sci Med 2008;67:1282–90.

7. Wooten J. Women as caregivers. J Womens Health 1998;7(5):597–9.

8. Johnson P, Chaboyer W, Foster M, et al. Caregivers of ICU patients discharged home: what burden do they face? Intensive Crit Care Nurs 2001;17:219–27.

9. Australian Bureau of Statistics (ABS). In: ABS Catalogue # 4430.0. Canberra: Government Printers; 1999 (booklet).

10. Tang Y, Chen S. Health promotion behaviors in Chinese family caregivers of patients with stroke. Health Promot Int 2002;17:329–39.

11. Huang C, Sousa V, Perng S, et al. Stressors, social support, depressive symptoms and general health status of Taiwanese caregivers of persons with stroke or Alzheimer's disease. J Clin Nurs 2009;18:502–11.

12. Pawasarat J. Barriers to employment: NSAF findings on preschool children, mothers' employment status and child care choices. National Survey of America's Families, U.S. Child Care Choices 1997 and 1999. Available at: http://2224.uwm. edu/eti/barriers/nsafus.htm. Accessed April 10, 2009.

13. Gornick J, Meyers M. Families that work: policies for reconciling parenthood and employment. New York: Russell Sage Foundation; 2003.

14. Wuest J, Hodgins M, Malcolm J, et al. The effects of past relationship and obligation on health and health promotion in women caregivers of adult family members. ANS Adv Nurs Sci 2007;30(3):206–20.

15. Cranswick K. Canada's caregivers. In: Canadian social trends. Ottawa, Ontario: Statistics Canada, #11-008-XPE; 1997 (booklet).

16. Morgan D, Semchuk K, Stewart N, et al. Rural families caring for a relative with dementia: barriers to use of formal services. Soc Sci Me 2002;55:1129–42.

17. Kim J. Dementia care in Korea: a case study of need. Dementia: The International Journal of Social Research and Practice 2002;1:135–9.

18. Kim S, Kim J, Stewart R, et al. Correlates of caregiver burden for Korean elders according to cognitive and functional status. Int J Geriatr Psychiatry 2006;21: 853–61.

19. Barecki-Gisolf J, Lucke J, Hockey R, et al. Transitions into informal caregiving and out of paid employment of women in their 50s. Soc Sci Med 2008;67:122–7.

20. Hochschild A. The second shift: working parents and the revolution at home. New York: Viking; 1989.

21. Lundberg U, Frankenhauser M. Stress and workload of men and women in high-ranking positions. J Occup Health Psychol 1999;4(2):142–51.

22. Tarimo E, Kohi T, Outwater A, et al. Gender roles and informal care for patients with AIDS: a qualitative study from an urban area in Tanzania. J Transcult Nurs 2009;20(1):61–8.

23. Montgomery R, Williams K. Implications of differential impacts of care-giving for future research on Alzheimer care. Aging Ment Health 2001;5:S23–34.

24. Sanders S. Is the glass half empty or full? Reflections on strain and gain in care-givers of individuals with Alzheimer disease. Soc Work Health Care 2005;40: 57–73.

25. Given B, Sherwood P. Family care for the older person with cancer. Semin Oncol Nurs 2006;22:43–50.

26. Aneshensel C, Pearlin L, Mullan J, et al. Profiles in caregiving: the unexpected career. San Diego (CA): The Academic Press; 1995.

27. Brodarty H, Hadzi-Pavlovic D. Psychosical effects on carers of living with persons with dementia. Aust N Z J Psychiatry 1990;24:351–61.

28. Elliott K, Campbell R. Changing ideas about family care for the elderly in Japan. J Cross Cult Gerontol 1993;8:119–35.

29. Holicky R. Caring for the caregivers: the hidden victims of illness and disability. Rehabil Nurs 1996;21(5):247–52.

30. Franzen-Dahlin A, Larson J, Murray V, et al. Predictors of psychological health in spouses of persons affected by stroke. J Clin Nurs 2007;16(5):885–91.

31. Pinquart M, Sorensen S. Differences between caregivers and noncaregivers in psychological health and physical health: a meta-analysis. Psychol Aging 2003;18(2):250–67.

32. Kosberg J, Cairl R. The cost of care index: a case management tool for screening informal care providers. Gerontologist 1986;26:273–85.

33. Zarit S, Reever K, Bach-Petersen J. Relatives of the impaired elderly: correlates of feelings of burden. Gerontol 1980;20:649–55.

34. Bedini L, Guinan D. "If I could just be selfish." Caregivers' perceptions of their entitlements to leisure. Leisure Sciences 1996;18:227–39.

35. Lee C, Gramotnev H. Transitions into and out of caregiving: health and social characteristics of mid-age Australian women. Psychol Health 2007;22(2): 193–209.

36. Ostwald S. Who is caring for the caregiver? Promoting spousal caregiver's health. Fam Community Health 2009;32(1S):S5–14.

37. Cutler L, Garner M. Reducing relocations stress after discharge from the inten-sive therapy unit. Intensive Crit Care Nurs 1995;11:333–5.

38. Bugge C, Alexander H, Hagen S. Stroke patients' informal caregivers: patient, caregiver, and service factors that affect caregiver strain. Stroke 1999;30: 1517–23.

39. Gillis C. Reducing family stress during and after coronary bypass surgery. Nurs Clin North Am 1984;19(1):103–11.

40. Davies N. Carers' opinions and emotional responses following cardiac surgery: cardiac rehabilitation implications for critical care nurses. Intensive Crit Care Nurs 2000;16:66–75.

41. Kipp W. Factors associated with the self-reported health status of female care-givers of AIDS patients. West J Nurs Res 2007;20(10):1–14.

42. Pinquart M, Sorensen S. Correlates of physical health of informal caregivers: a meta-analysis. J Gerontol B Psychol Sci Soc Sci 2007;62(2):P126–37.

43. Hirst M. Caring-related inequalities in psychological distress in Britain during the 1990s. J Public Health Med 2003;25:336–43.

44. Hirst M. Caregiver distress: a prospective, population-based study. Soc Sci Med 2005;61:697–708.

45. Singleton N, Maunt N, Cowie A, et al. Mental health of caregivers. London: The Stationery Office; 2002.

46. Bertrand R, Fredman L, Saczynski J. Are all caregivers created equal? Stress in caregivers to adults with and without dementia. J Aging Health 2006;18:534–51.

47. Zunzunegui M, Beland F, Llacer A, et al. Family, religion, and depressive symptoms in caregivers of disabled elderly. J Epidemiol Community Health 1999;53:364–9.
48. Schulz R, O'Brien A, Bookwala J, et al. Psychiatric and physical morbidity effects of dementia caregiving: prevalence, correlates, and causes. Gerontologist 1995;35:771–91.
49. Vitaliano P, Zhang J, Scanlan J. Is caregiving hazardous for one's physical health? a meta-analysis. Psychol Bull 2003;129:946–72.
50. Patterson T, Grant I. Interventions for caregiving in dementia: physical outcomes. Current Opinion in Psychiatry 2003;16:629–33.
51. DeFrias C, Tukko H, Rosenberg T. Caregiver physical and mental health predicts reactions to caregiving. Aging Ment Health 2005;9:331–6.
52. Murphy N, Christian B, Caplin D, et al. The health of caregivers for children with disabilities: caregiver perspectives. Child Care Health Dev 2006;33(2):180–7.
53. Schulz R, Beach S. Caregiving as a risk factor for mortality: the Caregiver Health Effects Study. JAMA 1999;282:2215–9.
54. Schulz R, Martire L. Family caregiving of persons with dementia: prevalence, health effects, and support strategies. Am J Geriatr Psychiatry 2004;12:240–9.
55. Reinhard S, Rosswurm M, Robinson K. Policy recommendations for family caregiver support. J Gerontol Nurs 2000;26(1):47–9.
56. Crosato K, Leipert B. Rural women caregivers in Canada. Rural Rem Health 2006;6:1–11.
57. Won C, Fitts S, Favaro S, et al. Community-based "powerful tools" intervention enhances health of caregivers. Arch Gerontol Geriatr 2008;46:89–100.

Index

Note: Page numbers of article titles are in **boldface** type.

A

Abortion services, normalizing into preventive framework in women's health care, 305–309
Adolescence, depression in girls during, 357–359
    promotion of women's health in, 283–284
    recommendations for HPV vaccines, 195–297
Adulthood, promotion of women's health in, 283–284
      chronic disease, 287
      irritable bowel syndrome, 285–286
      premenstrual syndrome, 284–285
      sleep disorders, 286
      vitamin D deficiency, 285
Advisory Committee on Immunization Practices, recommendations on HPV vaccine, 296
Advocacy, reproductive health, within the nursing profession, 311–312
Anxiety, depression and, in women, **355–364**
    comorbidity with somatic illness, 361–363
    in childhood and adolescence, 357–359
    menstruation, pregnancy, and menopause-related, 359–361

B

BRCA testing, as exemplar for genetic health care, 330–334
      decision making and, 332–334
      genes are passed down, 331–332
      genetics are familial, 331
Breast cancer, genetics of, **327–338**
      BRCA testing as exemplar for genetic health care, 330–334
        decision making and, 332–334
        genes are passed down, 331–332
        genetics are familial, 331
      guidelines for testing and management of genetic risk, 328–329
      hereditary breast cancer, 327–328
      risk across the life span, 329–330
Burden, of caregiving, on global women's health, 378–379

C

Cancer, breast cancer, genetics of, **327–338**
    effectiveness of computer-mediated patient education interventions, 349–350
      recurrent ovarian cancer, 350
Cardiac health. *See* Cardiovascular disease *and* Heart disease.
Cardiovascular disease, anxiety and depression comorbidity with, 361–362

Nurs Clin N Am 44 (2009) 385–392
doi:10.1016/S0029-6465(09)00064-4
0029-6465/09/$ – see front matter © 2009 Elsevier Inc. All rights reserved.

nursing.theclinics.com

Moving?

Make sure your subscription moves with you!

To notify us of your new address, find your **Clinics Account Number** (located on your mailing label above your name), and contact customer service at:

Email: journalscustomerservice-usa@elsevier.com

800-654-2452 (subscribers in the U.S. & Canada)
314-447-8871 (subscribers outside of the U.S. & Canada)

Fax number: 314-447-8029

Elsevier Health Sciences Division
Subscription Customer Service
3251 Riverport Lane
Maryland Heights, MO 63043

*To ensure uninterrupted delivery of your subscription, please notify us at least 4 weeks in advance of move.

ELSEVIER